IET CONTROL, ROBOTICS AND SENSORS SERIES 105

Mechatronic Hands

Other volumes in this series:

Volume 8 **A History of Control Engineering, 1800–1930** S. Bennett
Volume 18 **Applied Control Theory, 2nd Edition** J.R. Leigh
Volume 20 **Design of Modern Control Systems** D.J. Bell, P.A. Cook and N. Munro (Editors)
Volume 28 **Robots and Automated Manufacture** J. Billingsley (Editor)
Volume 33 **Temperature Measurement and Control** J.R. Leigh
Volume 34 **Singular Perturbation Methodology in Control Systems** D.S. Naidu
Volume 35 **Implementation of Self-tuning Controllers** K. Warwick (Editor)
Volume 37 **Industrial Digital Control Systems, 2nd Edition** K. Warwick and D. Rees (Editors)
Volume 39 **Continuous Time Controller Design** R. Balasubramanian
Volume 40 **Deterministic Control of Uncertain Systems** A.S.I. Zinober (Editor)
Volume 41 **Computer Control of Real-time Processes** S. Bennett and G.S. Virk (Editors)
Volume 42 **Digital Signal Processing: Principles, devices and applications** N.B. Jones and J.D.McK. Watson (Editors)
Volume 44 **Knowledge-based Systems for Industrial Control** J. McGhee, M.J. Grimble and A. Mowforth (Editors)
Volume 47 **A History of Control Engineering, 1930–1956** S. Bennett
Volume 49 **Polynomial Methods in Optimal Control and Filtering** K.J. Hunt (Editor)
Volume 50 **Programming Industrial Control Systems Using IEC 1131-3** R.W. Lewis
Volume 51 **Advanced Robotics and Intelligent Machines** J.O. Gray and D.G. Caldwell (Editors)
Volume 52 **Adaptive Prediction and Predictive Control** P.P. Kanjilal
Volume 53 **Neural Network Applications in Control** G.W. Irwin, K. Warwick and K.J. Hunt (Editors)
Volume 54 **Control Engineering Solutions: A practical approach** P. Albertos, R. Strietzel and N. Mort (Editors)
Volume 55 **Genetic Algorithms in Engineering Systems** A.M.S. Zalzala and P.J. Fleming (Editors)
Volume 56 **Symbolic Methods in Control System Analysis and Design** N. Munro (Editor)
Volume 57 **Flight Control Systems** R.W. Pratt (Editor)
Volume 58 **Power-plant Control and Instrumentation: The control of boilers and HRSG systems** D. Lindsley
Volume 59 **Modelling Control Systems Using IEC 61499** R. Lewis
Volume 60 **People in Control: Human factors in control room design** J. Noyes and M. Bransby (Editors)
Volume 61 **Nonlinear Predictive Control: Theory and practice** B. Kouvaritakis and M. Cannon (Editors)
Volume 62 **Active Sound and Vibration Control** M.O. Tokhi and S.M. Veres
Volume 63 **Stepping Motors, 4th Edition** P.P. Acarnley
Volume 64 **Control Theory, 2nd Edition** J.R. Leigh
Volume 65 **Modelling and Parameter Estimation of Dynamic Systems** J.R. Raol, G. Girija and J. Singh
Volume 66 **Variable Structure Systems: From principles to implementation** A. Sabanovic, L. Fridman and S. Spurgeon (Editors)
Volume 67 **Motion Vision: Design of compact motion sensing solution for autonomous systems** J. Kolodko and L. Vlacic
Volume 68 **Flexible Robot Manipulators: Modelling, simulation and control** M.O. Tokhi and A.K.M. Azad (Editors)
Volume 69 **Advances in Unmanned Marine Vehicles** G. Roberts and R. Sutton (Editors)
Volume 70 **Intelligent Control Systems Using Computational Intelligence Techniques** A. Ruano (Editor)
Volume 71 **Advances in Cognitive Systems** S. Nefti and J. Gray (Editors)
Volume 72 **Control Theory: A guided tour, 3rd Edition** J. R. Leigh
Volume 73 **Adaptive Sampling with Mobile WSN** K. Sreenath, M.F. Mysorewala, D.O. Popa and F.L. Lewis
Volume 74 **Eigenstructure Control Algorithms: Applications to aircraft/rotorcraft handling qualities design** S. Srinathkumar
Volume 75 **Advanced Control for Constrained Processes and Systems** F. Garelli, R.J. Mantz and H. De Battista
Volume 76 **Developments in Control Theory towards Glocal Control** L. Qiu, J. Chen, T. Iwasaki and H. Fujioka (Editors)
Volume 77 **Further Advances in Unmanned Marine Vehicles** G.N. Roberts and R. Sutton (Editors)
Volume 78 **Frequency-Domain Control Design for High-Performance Systems** J. O'Brien
Volume 80 **Control-oriented Modelling and Identification: Theory and practice** M. Lovera (Editor)
Volume 81 **Optimal Adaptive Control and Differential Games by Reinforcement Learning Principles** D. Vrabie, K. Vamvoudakis and F. Lewis
Volume 83 **Robust and Adaptive Model Predictive Control of Nonlinear Systems** M. Guay, V. Adetola and D. DeHaan
Volume 84 **Nonlinear and Adaptive Control Systems** Z. Ding
Volume 88 **Distributed Control and Filtering for Industrial Systems** M. Mahmoud
Volume 89 **Control-based Operating System Design** A. Leva *et al.*
Volume 90 **Application of Dimensional Analysis in Systems Modelling and Control Design** P. Balaguer
Volume 91 **An Introduction to Fractional Control** D. Valério and J. Costa
Volume 92 **Handbook of Vehicle Suspension Control Systems** H. Liu, H. Gao and P. Li
Volume 93 **Design and Development of Multi-Lane Smart Electromechanical Actuators** F.Y. Annaz
Volume 94 **Analysis and Design of Reset Control Systems** Y. Guo, L. Xie and Y. Wang
Volume 95 **Modelling Control Systems Using IEC 61499, 2nd Edition** R. Lewis & A. Zoitl
Volume 96 **Cyber-Physical System Design with Sensor Networking Technologies** S. Zeadally and N. Jabeur (Editors)

Mechatronic Hands

Prosthetic and Robotic Design

Paul H. Chappell

The Institution of Engineering and Technology

Published by the Institution of Engineering and Technology, London, United Kingdom

The Institution of Engineering and Technology is registered as a Charity in England & Wales (no. 211014) and Scotland (no. SC038698).

First published 2016

The Institution of Engineering and Technology
Michael Faraday House
Six Hills Way, Stevenage
Herts, SG1 2AY, United Kingdom

www.theiet.org

British Library Cataloguing in Publication Data
A catalogue record for this product is available from the British Library

ISBN 978-1-78561-154-4 (hardback)
ISBN 978-1-78561-155-1 (PDF)

Typeset in India by MPS Limited
Printed in the UK by CPI Group (UK) Ltd, Croydon

To Roma, Edward, Jonathan, Kate and Rowan

Contents

Acknowledgements

I am grateful to Rachel Hunt, House and Collections Manager, Cotehele (National Trust),[1] for showing me the hand displayed in the Hall, the hand replica and permitting me to take photographs of the House and hands.

Thanks are also due to all the PhD students from Electronics and Computer Science (and the former Department of Electrical Engineering) who have been awarded their degrees by the University of Southampton in the subject area of this book.

I wish to acknowledge Professor Peter J. Kyberd for his long standing research and interest in the subject of artificial hands; Peter, many thanks for all the debates and discussions we have had over the years.

I am grateful to Professor Neil M. White and Dr Andy Cranny for introducing me to sensor technology and for their enthusiasm about the design of hands and the integration of different sensors.

Without the technical support of some very skilled people, none of the hands made at the University of Southampton would have come to fruition. Thanks are due to all the technicians past and present, in the mechanical workshop and teaching laboratories, especially Mark Long, Barry Bailey and Richard Howell.

Thanks are due to Dr Cheryl Metcalf for promoting the Southampton Hand Assessment Procedure.

[1]Cotehele House, St. Dominick, Saltash, Cornwall, PL12 6TA, UK

Preface

A motivation for writing this book is to gather together the accumulated knowledge about artificial hands that has been gained at Southampton over several decades. This research was started by the late Professor James (Jim) M. Nightingale in the 1960s. He once said to me that we (he) had not published much about artificial hands for the disabled. Hopefully this book will to some extent correct this omission. I have often been asked by undergraduate and postgraduate students about the design of artificial hands. They will now be able to consult this book and gain an insight into the range of technologies that are needed in the construction of a working hand. Mechanical components obviously form the structure of any hand while there are some lesser known ideas that need to be explored such as how to process a slip signal.

In 1952, at an international conference attended by 2000 surgeons, held in Madrid, there was concern that an artificial device should be easy to use. In the report by Time Magazine, engineers were studying the use of sensors, albeit six simple pressure switches attached to the stump of an amputee. A photograph from this Time Magazine article shows a person fitted with an artificial arm. It appears in one of the 46 colour screen prints call 'Bunk' made by Sir Eduardo Paolopzzi in 1972 which is how I came across the photograph in the National Art Gallery, Sydney, Australia. It is probably still true that better sensors with good characteristics such as low power consumption and small size are needed to realise the aim of making a user-friendly device. This aspect is even more prevalent with modern hands that have multiple actuators and degrees of freedom. A latest commercial design claims 36 different types of grip. The selection and coordination of these grips needs careful consideration and the assistance of an electronic digital system. Also the use of position sensors, to measure the position of each finger and thumb, can be used in an electronic controller to avoid mechanical interference between them and the accidental clashing and locking of fingers and thumb.

A degree in the physical sciences will aid in an understanding of the analytical parts of the book or more specifically an engineering degree; mechanical, electrical or electronic. The subject areas of control theory, circuit theory, electronics, mechanics, materials and basic mathematics are needed. The desire to make an artificial hand anthropomorphic with natural movements and connected directly into the nervous system requires a study of human anatomy and physiology; bones of the hand wrist and elbow, their joints and muscles and the nervous system.

The book is intended to illustrate the technical design characteristics of the main components that go into forming an artificial hand whether it is a simple design that does not have a natural appearance or a more complicated design where there are multiple movements of the fingers and thumb. It could be used as an undergraduate text for final year or Master of Science degrees in a medical engineering or robotics course.

List of Symbols

a	Area (m^3), proportion of a link (mm) and data
a_i	ith weight of averaging process
A	Amplitude, end of link l_2 , velocity constant, gain, constant, constant acceleration
A_1	Constant
A_2	Constant
A_3	Constant
A'	Axis label
b	Proportion of a link (mm) and data
$\mathbf{B}$	Magnetic field (T)
B	End of link l_1, friction constant
c	data
C	Capacitance (F), end of link l_2
C_f	Feedback capacitance (F)
C_p	Piezoelectric sensor capacitance (F)
d	Data sample, dimension of surface pattern (mm) and diameter (cm)
$\bar{d}$	mean of data
D	end of link s_1'
d_1, d_{20}	data samples 1 to 20
d_e	Euclidean distance
d_i	ith sample
d_j	jth sample
D_{n1}	N_1 diode
D_{n2}	N_2 diode
D_{p1}	P_1 diode
D_{p2}	P_2 diode
d_{sj}	j^{th} digital signal (either 0 or 1)
e	Error and data

E	End of link l_1' and energy
e_k	Kinetic energy
e_p	Potential energy
$\boldsymbol{f}$	Force (N)
f	Function, scalar force (N), data and frequency (Hz)
f_a to f_d	Forces from four sensors and accelerometer functions
F	End of link l_2'
f_R	Reaction force (N)
f_x	Force in the x direction (N)
f_z	Force in the z direction (N)
F	Grip force and end of link s_2'
F_m	Tension in the drive belt between the middle and distal phalanges (N)
F_p	Tension in the drive belt between the palm and middle phalanges (N)
F_t	Force normal to the distal phalange; fingertip force (N)
g	Acceleration due to the Earth's gravitational field, gram and data
$G(s)$	Motor transfer function
G_r	Gearbox ratio
h	Data
$H(s)$	Feedback transfer function
i	Current (A), data and index
i_a	Armature current (A)
i_p	Piezoelectric sensor current (A)
j	Index and data
J	moment of inertia (kg m^2) and joule
k	Constant
K_d	Derivative constant of PID
k_e	Elastic constant ($N \cdot m^{-1}$)
K_i	Integral constant of PID
k_m	Back emf constant
k_o	Closed-loop gain
K_p	Position sensor gain, proportional constant of PID
l	Length (m)
l_d	Length of distal phalange (mm)
l_f	Length of finger (m)

l_m	Length of middle phalange (mm)
l_p	Length of proximal phalange (mm)
l_1 to l_3	Links of the four-bar mechanism (mm)
$l_1^{'}, l_2^{'}$	Links of the second four-bar mechanism (mm)
L	Inductance (H)
L_a	Armature inductance (H)
meanvar	Mean variance
m	Mass, measured variable
M	Number of windows
n	Number of samples
nat	Unit of entropy or information
N_1	N-channel MOSFET
N_2	N-channel MOSFET
O	Origin of four-bar mechanism
p_i	Probability of *i*th value
P	External force (N)
P_0	Precision posture
P_1	P-channel MOSFET and precision posture
P_2	P-channel MOSFET and precision posture
q	Electron charge, 1.6×10^{-19} (C)
r	Resistance (Ω)
r_d	Radius of distal pulley (mm)
r_{m1}	Radius of input middle pulley (mm)
r_{m2}	Radius of output middle pulley (mm)
r_p	Radius of proximal pulley (mm)
r_t	Distance from axis of proximal pulley to fingertip (mm)
r_1 and r_2	Distances between pivots of the four-bar mechanism
R	Resistance (Ω) and reaction force (N)
R_a	Armature resistance and circuit resistance (Ω)
R_b	Motor gearbox ratio
R_f	Feedback resistance (Ω)
R_o	Parameter of an FSR (Ω)
R_{sg}	Strain gauge resistance (Ω)
R_{sgl}	Lower strain gauge resistance (Ω)
R_{sgl1}	First lower strain gauge resistance (Ω)
R_{sgl2}	Second lower strain gauge resistance (Ω)

R_{sgu}	Upper strain gauge resistance (Ω)
R_{sgu1}	First upper strain gauge resistance (Ω)
R_{sgu2}	Second upper strain gauge resistance (Ω)
R_{ww}	Worm-wheel ratio
R^2	Coefficient of determination
R_1	AC amplifier input resistor (Ω)
R_2	AC amplifier feedback resistor (Ω)
s	Laplace transform variable and signal
$s(i)$	Signal at time interval, i
S_o	Initial value of exponential decay
s_a	Accelerometer output signal from device a
s_b	Accelerometer output signal from device b
s_c	Accelerometer output signal from device c
s_1, s_2	Links of the four-bar mechanism
s_1', s_2'	Links of the second four-bar mechanism
sm_3	$(r_2+s_2+l_2)/2$, expression for the four-bar mechanism
sm_5	$(r_2+s_2+l_2)/2$, expression for the four-bar mechanism
sm_7	$(r_2+s_1+l_1)/2$, expression for the four-bar mechanism
sm_8	$(r_1+s_2+l_1)/2$, expression for the four-bar mechanism
sm_{25}	$(r_2+s_1+l_1)/2$, expression for the four-bar mechanism
S_1	Parameter of an FSR ($Sm \cdot N^{-1}$)
S_2	Parameter of an FSR (S)
t	Time (s)
t_k	Thickness (m)
t_{k0}	Thickness or separation for zero force (m)
t_0	Time at which slipping starts (s)
t_1	Time at which slipping ceases (s)
t_2	Slip end time (s)
t_j	Time for task j (s)
$\overline{t_{nj}}$	Mean time for normative group
t_r	Transmission ratio
T	Torque (N), fingertip, time to reach peak velocity
T_l	Load torque (N·m)
T_m	Motor torque (N)
T_p	Input torque (N)
T_{pp}	Torque at the proximal joint (N)

u	Input signal
v	Voltage (V), velocity ($mm \cdot s^{-1}$)
$\mathbf{v}$	Drift velocity ($m \cdot s^{-1}$)
var	Variance
var_i	ith variance
v_b	Back emf voltage
V_a	Supply voltage to a DC motor and input voltage
V_{in}	Input voltage (V)
v_o	Output voltage (V)
V_o	Output voltage (V)
V_{out}	Output voltage (V)
v_r	Relative velocity
v_s	Slip signal
V_z	Initial value of exponential decay at time $t = 0$
V_+	Positive supply voltage (V)
V_-	Negative supply voltage (V)
w	Width
W	Window length
x	Generic variable and coordinate
X	Peak velocity
$\ddot{x}$	Acceleration in the x direction
x_a	x-axis of a three axis accelerometer
x_{A}	x component of joint A in the four-bar mechanism
x_{B}	x component of joint B in the four-bar mechanism
x_{C}	x component of joint C in the four-bar mechanism
x_n	Slip distance at nth time interval
x_T	x component of fingertip in four-bar link
$x_{u\mathrm{BC}}$	Unit component of link BC in four-bar link
y	Variable and coordinate and slip distance
Y	Laplace transformed variable of y
$y(i)$	Absolute signal at time interval, i
$\overline{y(i)}$	Mean of the data $y(i)$
$\ddot{y}$	Acceleration in the y direction
y_a	y-axis of a three axis accelerometer
y_{A}	y component of joint A in the four-bar mechanism
y_{B}	y component of joint B in the four-bar mechanism

y_C	y component of joint C in the four-bar mechanism
y_T	y component of fingertip in four-bar linkage
y_{uBC}	Unit component of link BC in four-bar linkage
y_1	Starting position
y_2	End position
z	Variable, coordinate and statistical score
z_j	Score for the jth prehensile pattern
$\ddot{z}$	Acceleration in the z direction
z_a	z-axis of a three axis accelerometer
β	Angle with respect to the x-y plane
γ	Angle with respect to the z-y plane
ε	Strain and permittivity of a material
ε_o	Permittivity of free space
ε_r	Dielectric constant of a material
θ	Angle with respect to the x-z plane
θ_1', θ_9'	Angles of second four-bar linkage
θ_1 to θ_{16}	Angles of the four-bar linkage mechanisms
θ_{AC}	Angle of link AC
θ_{BC}	Angle of link BC
θ_i	Input angle
θ_o	Output angle
θ_r	Demanded finger position
μ	Coefficient of friction
ρ	Resistivity (Ωm)
σ_{nj}	Standard deviation of the normative group
τ_o	Closed loop time constant
ω	Frequency
ω_m	Angular velocity of motor
ω_{pp}	Angular velocity of proximal joint
Δ	Change in variable

Abbreviations

Abbreviation	Description
ABS	Acrylonitrile butadiene styrene
ADL	Activities of daily living
CMMR	Common mode rejection ratio
CNC	Computer numerical control
DARPA	Defence Advanced Research Projects Agency
ECG	Electrocardiogram
EM	Electromagnetic
EMC	Electromagnetic compatibility
EMG	Electromyographic
ENG	Electroneurograhpic
exp	Exponential, e^x
FFT	Fast Fourier Transform
LED	Light emitting diode
IC	Integrated circuit
IOF	Index of functionality
ln	Natural logarithm
MEMS	Micro-electro-mechanical systems
mNm	Millinewton metre
PLA	Polylactic acid or Polylactide
PTFE	Polytetrafluoroethylene
PID	Proportional, integral and derivative
R&D	Research and development
SAMS	Southampton Adaptive Manipulation Scheme
SHAP	Southampton Hand Assessment Procedure
UK	United Kingdom

Chapter 1
Introduction

This book is about the design of artificial hands for people, who through trauma or congenitally, only have one or no natural hands. It is not focused on robotics although there are naturally similarities between the design of a robotic hand and that for a limb replacement. A hand for an amputee may have sensors to detect force at the fingertips as will a hand for a robot. However, a major difference is that the mass of a prosthetic device for an adult should be limited to less than 500 g, and its physical size should be similar to that of a human hand. A hand for a child of 6 years should have a mass of less than 200 g. A prosthetic hand will be attached to the user's forearm by a customised socket which is placed over the residual limb. A heavy hand creates pressure points on the skin surface of the forearm and can be uncomfortable and unacceptable. The greater the mass of a hand, the more the muscles in the human arm have to work to move the hand about, putting strain on a person's shoulder and elbow. Robotic hands do not have to meet these particular requirements. Increasing the mass of a hand decreases the mass of the object that can held at the end of a robot arm but should not lead to the device being unusable. If the total mass at the end of an arm is too great, it will not move.

Graphical artists and the producers of science fiction films have created hands for humanoids and robots that appear to have superhuman strength and function. These media designs create the belief that people with science and technology degrees will make a hand that has capabilities beyond that of a natural hand and at the same time have the appearance of a natural hand. Surely if a super hand could be made then it would be compromised in some way, i.e., not be anthropomorphic or be too large. The basic laws of physics and chemistry are applicable to any design. Often something new is developed, and the media hype creates an incorrect impression of the capabilities of an artificial hand. The expectations of the new technology are not realised in practise, leading to dissatisfaction in the amputee population.

An artificial hand requires some means of control. This implies that the user can send information to the hand. The user inputs can be from mechanical straps attached to the shoulder as found in the split hook [1] or in an electronic form that is fed to an electronic controller (Figure 1.1). An actuator such as an electric motor moves a part of the mechanism, which could be the first finger for example. If the four fingers are controlled, then four motors could be used. Sensors mounted on or inside a hand can measure variables such as finger force or temperature.

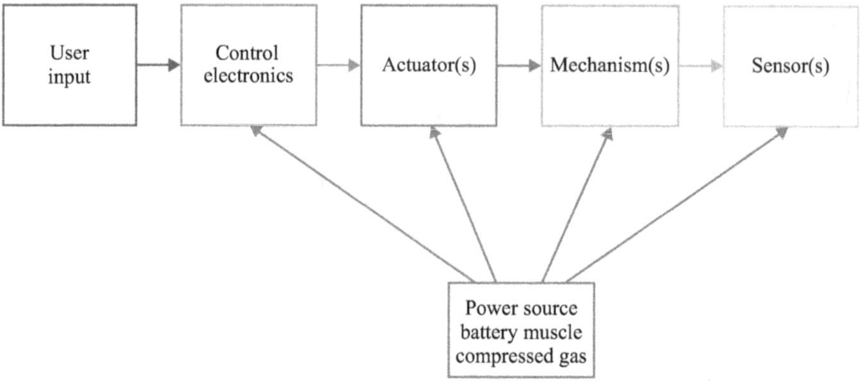

Figure 1.1 Block diagram showing components of an artificial hand

The signals from different types of sensors could be used to warn the user that maximum force has been generated or that a hot object has been touched for example. For movement of the mechanical parts to occur, a power source is needed which could be from a battery or from the human body, i.e., contraction of a skeletal muscle that is used in the split hook.

The text is written for a technical audience, in particular undergraduates, postgraduates and engineering designers. There are various types of hand such as a passive one that has no power source and is designed to have as natural an appearance as possible. A split hook is one that is powered from straps around the shoulders. However, this book focuses on powered hands that are controlled by the small electrical signals from residual muscles and are called myoelectric hands.

1.1 Brief history of artificial hands

This section focuses on two particular periods, i.e., the sixteenth century and the period of the two world wars. There is a wealth of material to be found in the literature that provides a fuller history of the development of artificial hands.

Research and Development (R&D) of the technology for artificial hands has typically coincided with major conflicts around the world when service personnel return from war with missing limbs or there are civilian casualties. During and after the First World War, replacement artificial limbs were made by a number of companies. In London, United Kingdom, some of the companies providing mechanical hands were J. & E. Ferris [2, 3], John Bell & Croyden [4], W. R. Grossmith Ltd. [5] and Hugh Steeper Ltd [6]. For example, W. R. Grossmith Ltd could supply a 'Light metal arm with fully articulated hand, controlled elbow joint, etc.' at a cost of £33 (about $50) [5]. These companies made a range of hands, wrists and forearms out of metals, plastics and leather that were cosmetic or had some gripping function to hold everyday objects. There were specialised accessories such as a combined knife and fork and one ironically was a gun rest.

In the introduction to their treatise on the manufacture of artificial limbs, J. & E. Ferris state:

> An Arm, such as is usually supplied, is simply an appendage, of which scarcely the slightest use can be made. With arms, having hands and fingers manufactured by us, many things, such as writing, drawing, painting, book-keeping, gardening, bicycle riding, working with a lathe, playing the violin, and much other work and pleasurable employment can, with a little patience and practice, be accomplished, and thus the artificial appliance becomes in the course of a short time not merely an ornamental member, but a most useful and reliable substitute [2, 3].

Some of these companies have ceased trading, while others have flourished, e.g., RSL Steeper Ltd.

In the United States of America, a program of R&D was started in 2006 by the Defence Advanced Research Projects Agency (DARPA) called 'Revolutionizing Prosthetics' [7]. Previous to this relatively recent upsurge of prosthetic design during the two world wars also provided the impetus to make better designs as did the congenital limb loss in the 1960s from the drug thalidomide.

Ambroise Paré (1510, Bourg-Hersent – 1590, Paris, France) is recognised as a pioneer in surgery and prosthetics [8–10]. He was appointed surgeon to the kings of France; Henry II, Francis II, Charles IX and Henry III. During his attendance to wounded soldiers, he invented the artificial hand shown in Figure 1.2. In his design are four cogs mounted in the palm at approximately the position of the

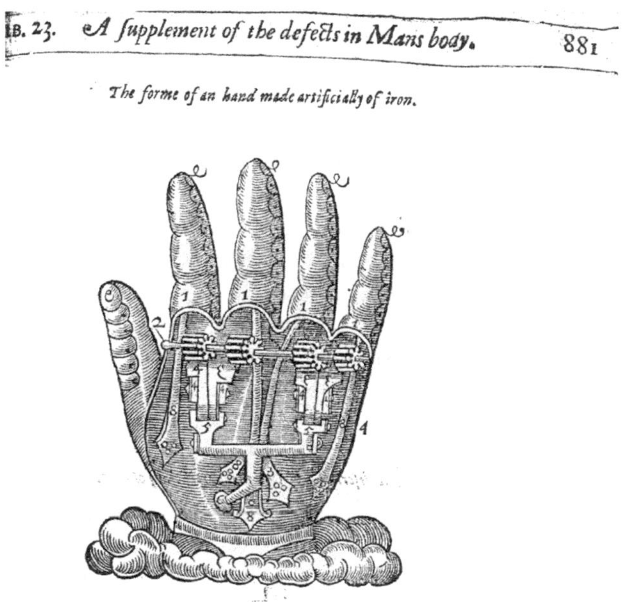

Figure 1.2 Design of a hand from the sixteenth century by Ambroise Paré 'The forme of a hand made artificially of iron'

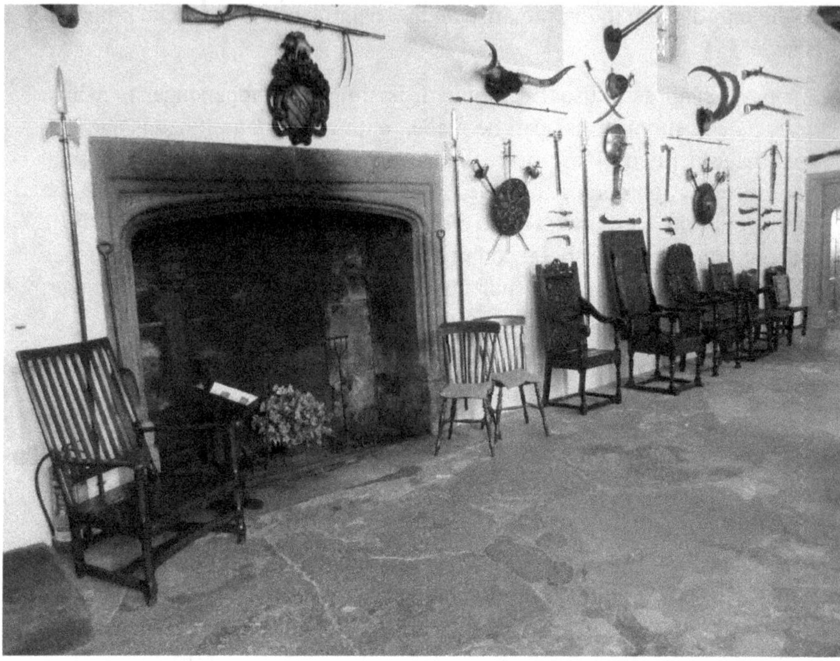

Figure 1.3 Entrance Hall at Cotehele. Notice the piece of armour hanging directly below the shield under the fifth chair from the left

metacarpal–phalangeal joints. There appears to be metal sheets connected to the cogs in the palm that are grouped in pairs; one set for the first and second fingers and one set for the third and fourth fingers.

I visited an outstanding Tudor house owned by the UK National Trust called Cotehele while on holiday in Cornwall. The main entrance to the house is from a courtyard into a magnificent Hall, which leads to the rooms of the building. After walking around and on returning to the Hall, I noticed among the armoury hanging on the wall an interesting article (Figures 1.3–1.5). What struck me was the similarity of the hand to the drawing that I had seen in a book some years earlier in the library of the Thackray Medical Museum in Becket Street, Leeds (Figure 1.2) especially the cogs located at the base of the fingers. Interestingly, the drawing and the actual prosthesis have the same handedness, i.e., a design for replacement of a left hand and are both sixteenth century. However, the arm in Cotehele possibly originates from France but was formerly thought to be Germany.

There are three levers arranged around the wrist. The two on the palmar side operate the fingers (Figure 1.6). Pulling the first lever which is nearest the thumb, releases the cogs of the first and second fingers (Figure 1.6). If not restrained, the fingers will flex into the palm under the spring action of metal strips inside the palm and fingers. The second lever operates the third and fourth fingers (Figure 1.7). Thus the spring and locking mechanisms are combined together. Each finger can be individually flexed (Figures 1.8–1.11). Notice that the metal in these figures looks

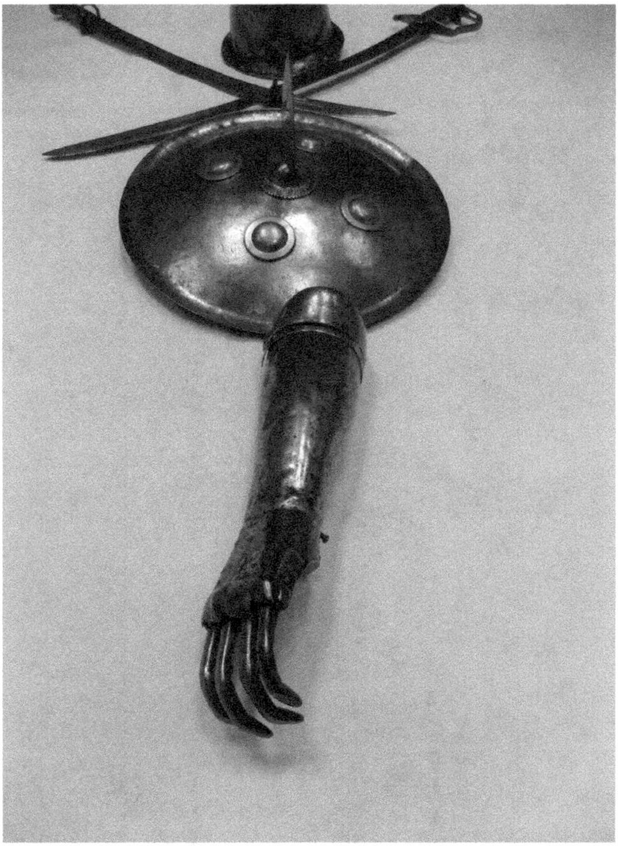

Figure 1.4 The forearm and hand hanging from the wall in the entrance Hall at Cotehele (mass 1.27 kg)

shiny compared to that in the previous figures. The reason for this change in appearance is because a replica of the ancient arm has been made by Context Engineering (Powys, Wales). The fingers can be flexed from fully extended (first position) and locked into three other positions (Figures 1.12–1.14). The replica of the forearm and hand has a mass of 1.63 kg.

A third lever located on the side of the wrist operates the thumb (Figure 1.5). The thumb is in the first position and fully extended in Figures (1.8–1.11). A further five positions allow for the thumb to be flexed into the palm (Figures 1.15–1.19).

The hand is remarkably versatile, allowing for a potential 1280 (5×4^4) combinations of finger and thumb positions and hence grips (Figures 1.20 and 1.21). However, when the thumb moves into either the third, fourth or fifth positions, it may clash with some flexed fingers reducing the number of practical combinations.

Further historical information can be found in an article by Childress, who has written an interesting account of powered limbs from the early twentieth century to the mid-1980s [11].

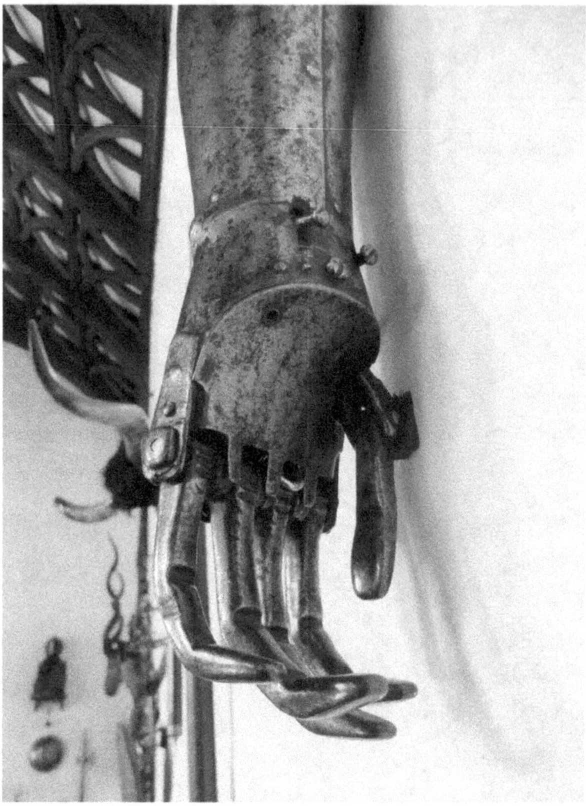

Figure 1.5 A view of the hand

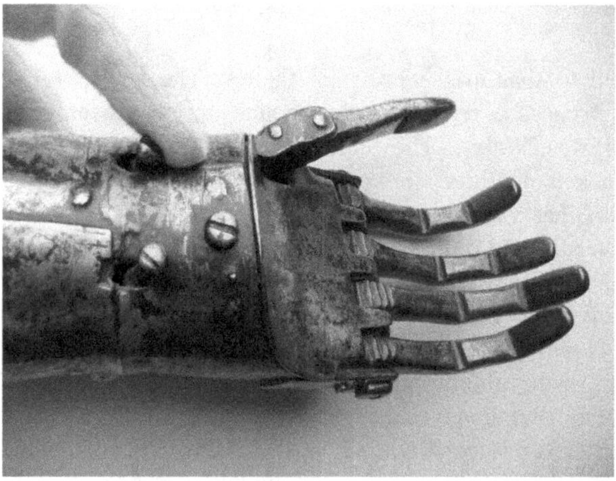

Figure 1.6 Palmar view of the hand showing the first release lever connected to two of the paws

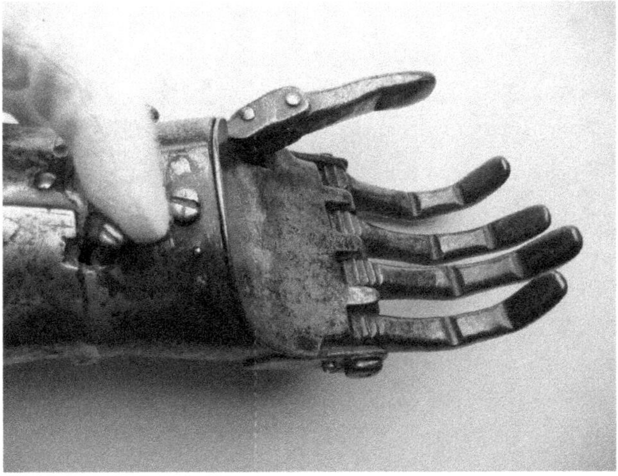

Figure 1.7 Palmar view of the hand showing the second release lever connected to two of the paws

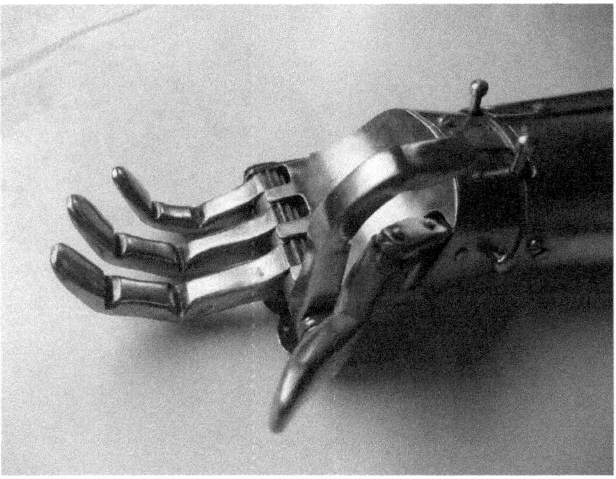

Figure 1.8 First finger flexion

1.2 Myoelectrically controlled hands

The first development of a hand controlled by myoelectric signals is attributed to Reinhold Reiter who was a student, studying physics in Munich in 1948 [12].

A myoelectrically controlled hand has many components in order to take electrical energy from a battery and convert it into mechanical energy to move fingers and a thumb and to grip an object. Figure 1.22 shows a block diagram of the

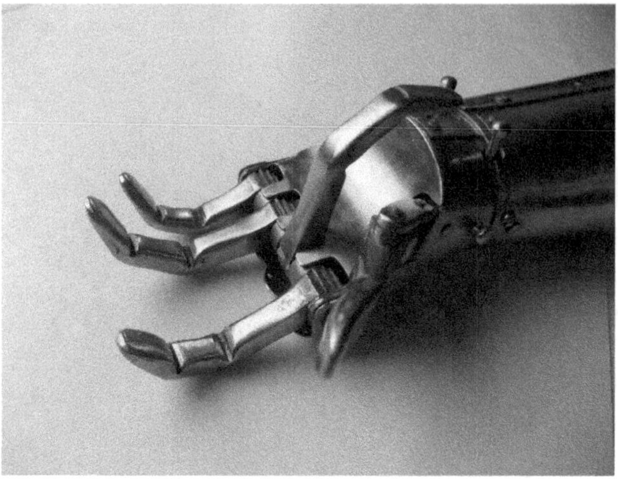

Figure 1.9 Second finger flexion

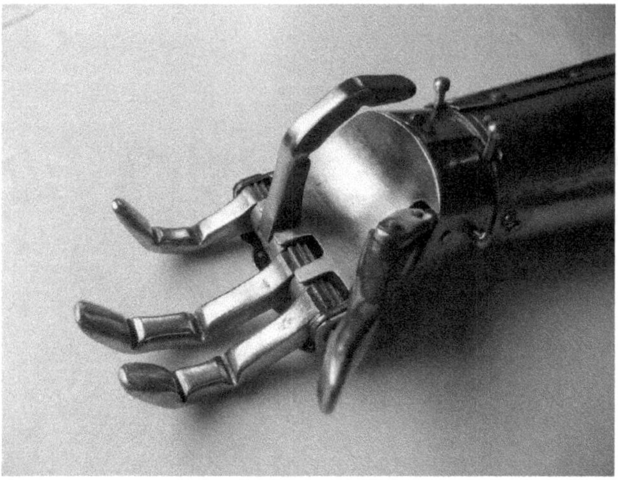

Figure 1.10 Third finger flexion

main parts. Electrodes attached to the skin surface detect small electrical signals called elecromyographical (EMG) signals. These have a very small magnitude of about 10 μV and need to be amplified. On contraction of a residual muscle that may be present in the stump of the forearm, the controller calculates the overall intensity of the signal and opens the hand. On relaxing the muscle, the signal strength falls and the hand will close. This arrangement is called voluntary opening as on relaxing the muscle, the hand automatically closes. Another method is where the hand is open and voluntary closing allows for the amputee to grip an object.

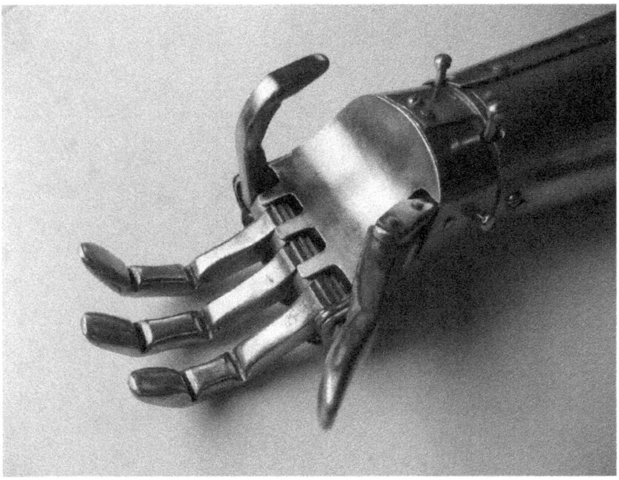

Figure 1.11 Fourth finger flexion

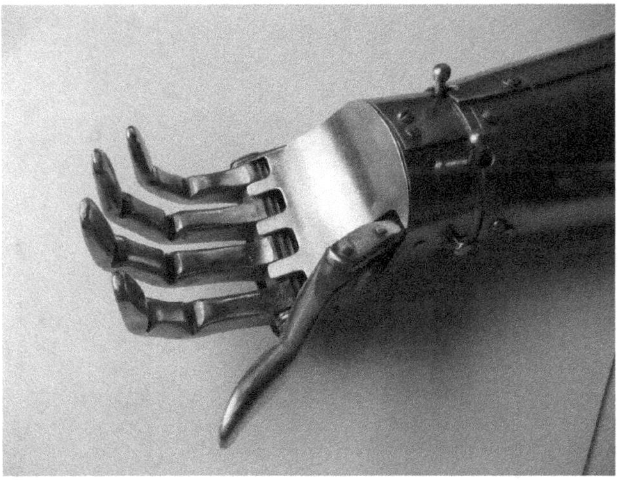

Figure 1.12 Flexion of the fingers into the second position

An open-loop system allows for little feedback of information about the grip force or finger position relative to the palmar surface. A gentle force cannot be accurately imparted to a delicate object such as a hen's egg to avoid excessive force. However, in lifting a heavy object such as a suitcase, maximum grip force can be generated, which results in the motor stalling and vibrating the finger mechanism. There vibrations can be felt through the residual stump giving feedback and confidence to the wearer that a secure grip has been achieved. In contrast, an electronically controlled feedback system (Figure 1.23) can provide a faster response and better control of finger position and grip force.

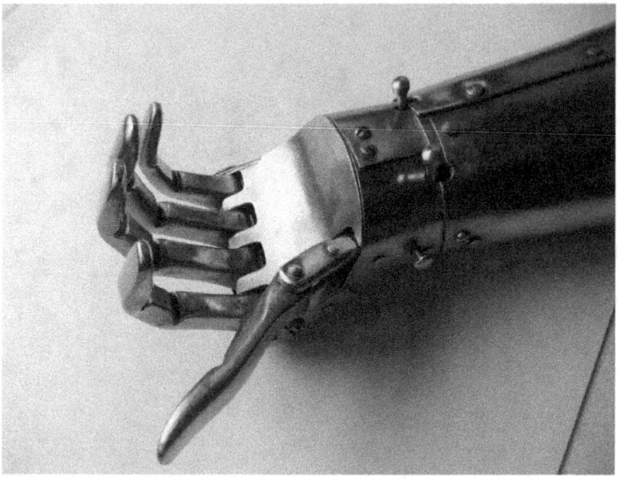

Figure 1.13 Flexion of the fingers into the third position

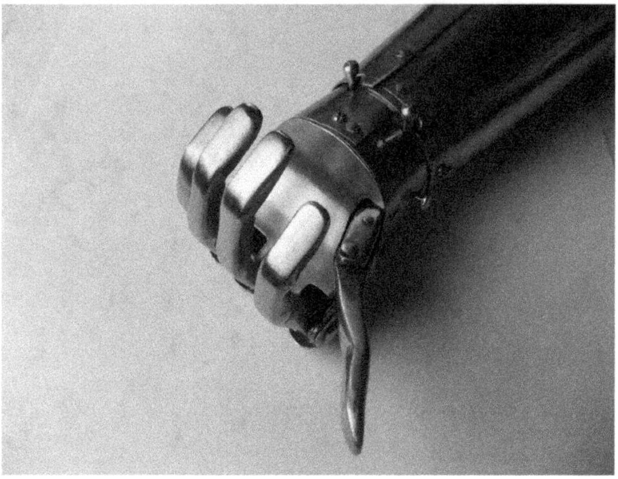

Figure 1.14 Full flexion of the fingers into the fourth position

1.3 Components

An artificial hand can have several components and these are listed below.

- mechanical structure (skeleton) to support the hand parts
- actuators to move the fingers and thumb
- sensors to provide information for an electronic controller and the user
- electronics that amplify signals from sensors and provide for an interface between the user and the actuators

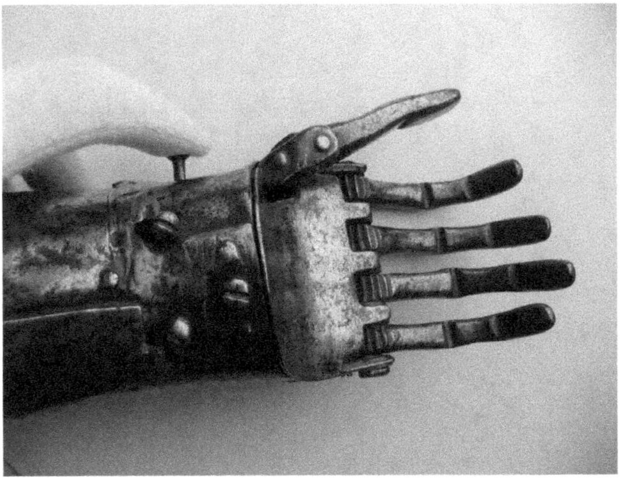

Figure 1.15 Release lever for the thumb

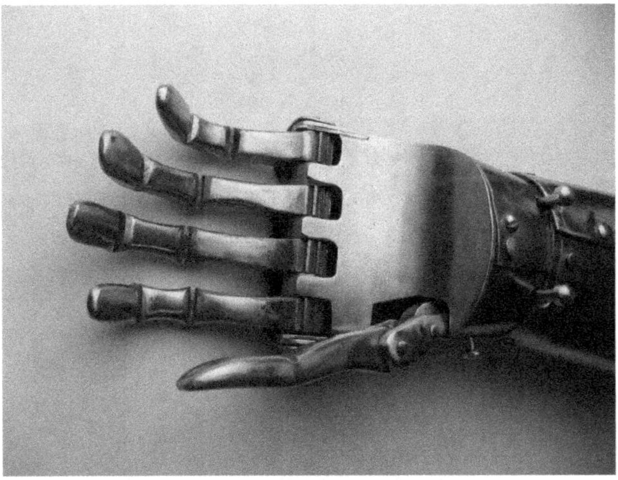

Figure 1.16 Second position of the thumb

- power source that is typically from rechargeable batteries
- an outer cosmetic glove called a cosmesis to protect the hand and provide good visual appearance
- a prosthetic socket to attach the hand to the user

Some components are not contained within the boundaries of the hand, e.g., batteries and the electronic controller are usually located away from the hand in the socket that attaches a hand to a person's stump. Power and electronic signals are transmitted through the mechanical wrist that contains a central plug and socket, so that a hand can be easily attached and removed from the socket.

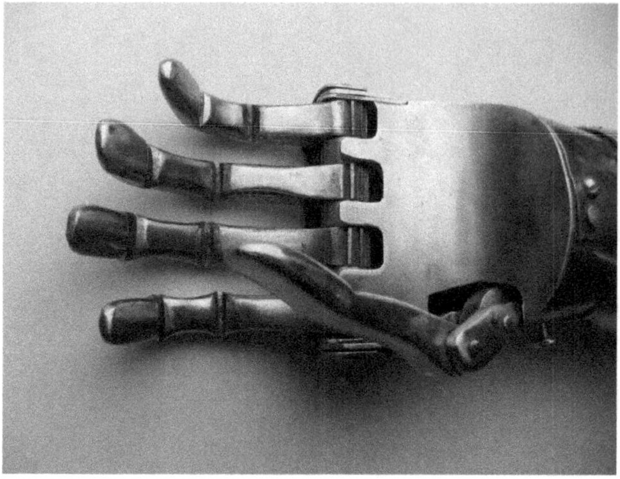

Figure 1.17 Third position of the thumb

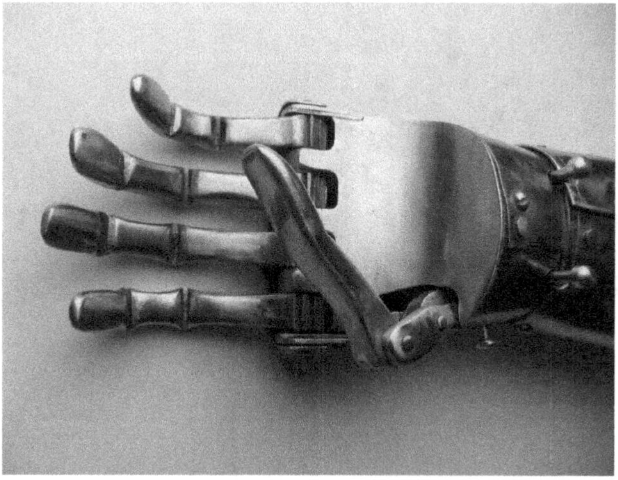

Figure 1.18 Fourth position of the thumb

Adding an extra component to a hand design may be considered as useful, but it will add mass and from a comfort perspective is undesirable. There has to be structural material to hold the components together, so there is very little that can be done to reduce mass here other than to consider making the hand from light-weight materials. It might be thought beneficial to add a further actuator in order to provide more degrees of freedom. But Figure 1.24 demonstrates that a high proportion of a total hand mass is from the actuators [13]. The design in Figure 1.24 is

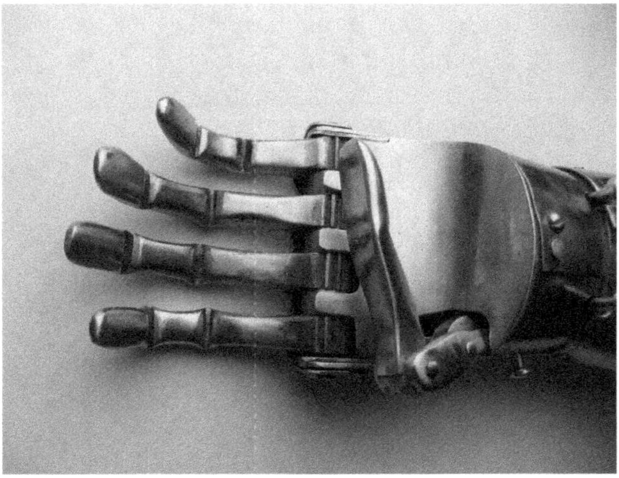

Figure 1.19 Fifth position of the thumb

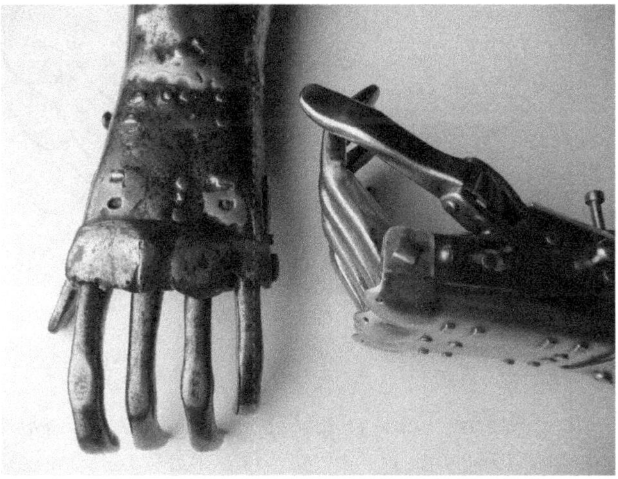

Figure 1.20 Ancient hand on the left and replica on the right where the thumb tip opposes the side of partially flexed first finger

based on six actuators and is made from carbon fibre composite for the structure [13]. The actuators account for over half the total mass. Figure 1.25 shows the mass breakdown without a glove where the thumb has two movements and is heavier than a single finger. The 17% for a single finger is further broken down in Figure 1.26, which demonstrates that the motor, gearbox and worm-wheel drive, which are the main components of the actuator, contribute to 69% of the total mass

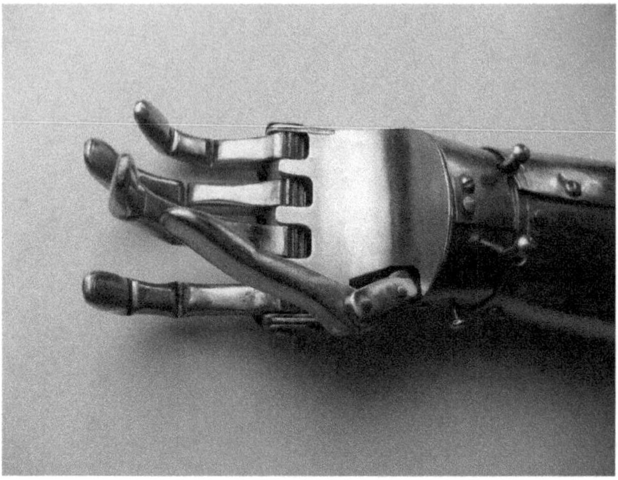

Figure 1.21 Partially flexed second finger in the second position opposing a partially flexed thumb in the third position

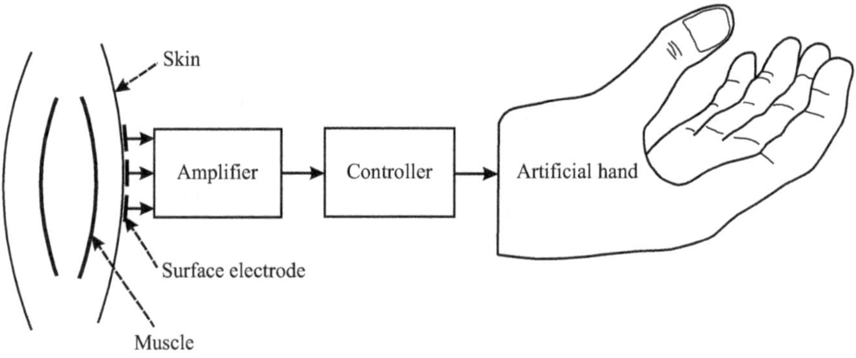

Figure 1.22 Block diagram of the typical open-loop control system for a myoelectric hand

of a finger. Fingertip forces of about 5 N are needed to hold most everyday objects. For a non-anthropomorphic hand the finger forces can be much larger at 150 N or more, but the compromise is to use just one powerful motor resulting in a reduction of the number of digit movements and functionality.

1.4 Mechanisms and actuators

An artificial hand can consist of simply a finger or group of fingers and a thumb driven by one actuator such as a DC motor and gearbox. The ridged finger and

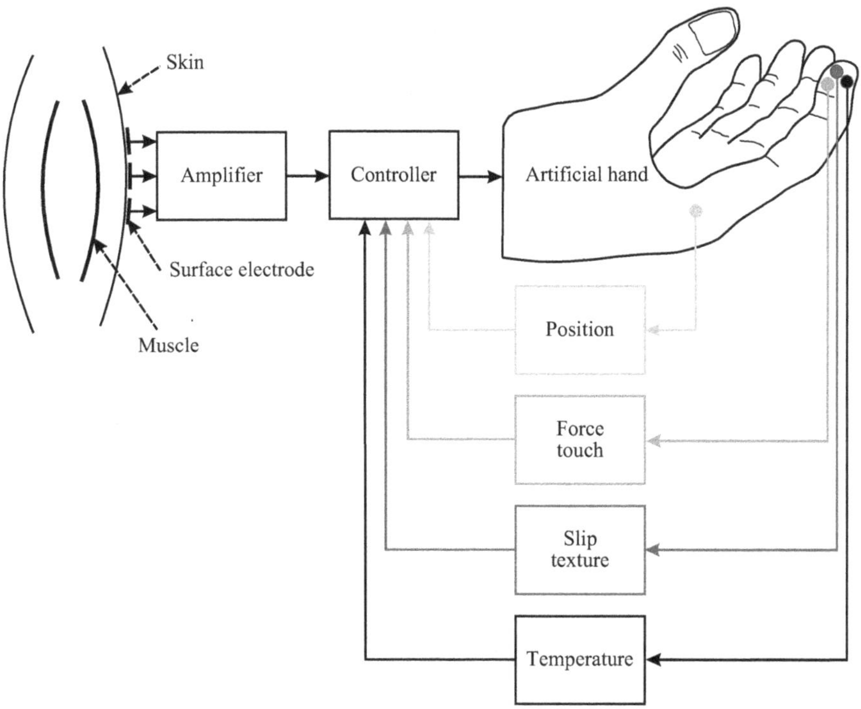

Figure 1.23 Closed-loop system with sensors shown for the first finger. Separate sensors are also needed for the thumb and other digits

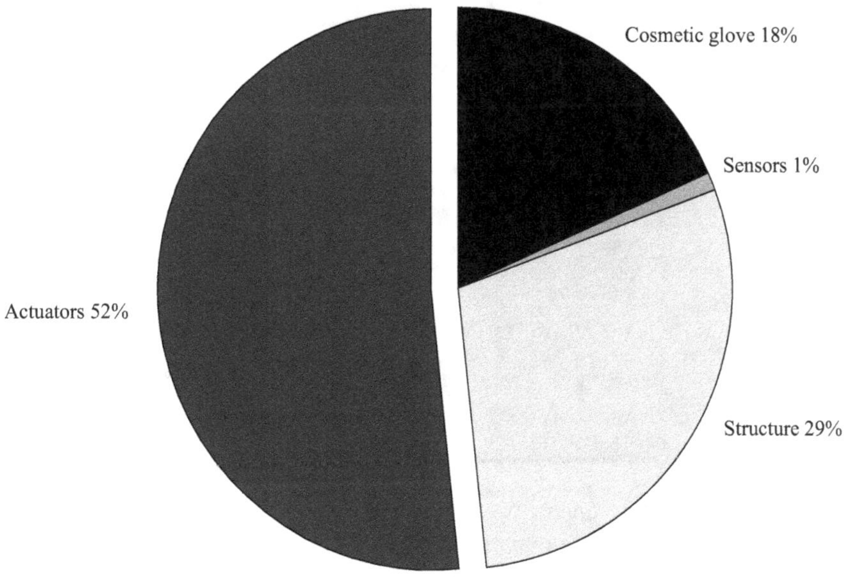

Figure 1.24 Mass distribution of a hand with six actuators including the glove but excluding the electronic controller, power source and socket [13]

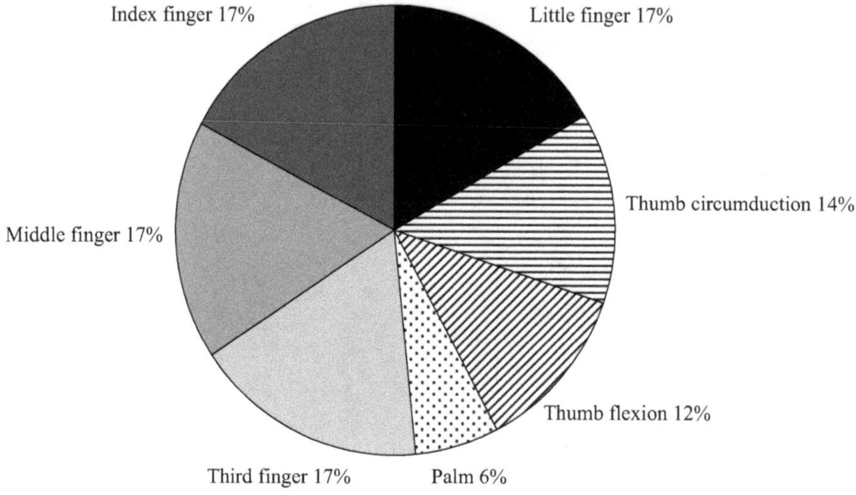

Figure 1.25 Mass distribution of a hand with four fingers and a thumb and six actuators [13]

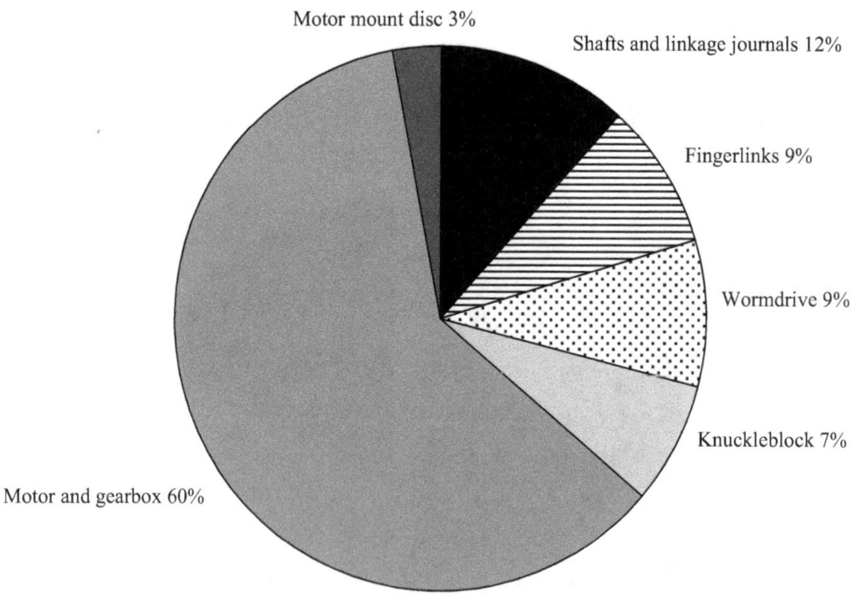

Figure 1.26 Mass distribution of the components in a single finger [13]

thumb are rotated about one or two axes to form a pinch grip at the tips. When a finger flexes into the palm, a more natural movement can be achieved with several linkages and pivots but at the expense of a loss of mechanical advantage. It is desirable for the fingers to move at a similar rate to natural fingers and thumb, but in an artificial mechanism, there is a trade-off between achieving a fast movement and high grip force.

1.5 Power sources

Any power source should have good properties. It should have high energy density ($J{\cdot}kg^{-1}$), low cost and hence easy availability, low maintenance and be safe in operation. The most widely used power source is electrical from rechargeable batteries. This choice provides a convenient high energy density and is quiet in use. Battery development for small devices benefits the prosthetic market, and there are several technologies that provide enough stored energy for the use of an artificial hand over 1 day. For example, a nickel–metal–hydride battery pack operating at 6 V has a typical energy density of 0.2 $MJ{\cdot}kg^{-1}$. It has a mass of 72 g and a volume of 4700 mm^3 ($10 \times 10 \times 45$ mm). It can provide a maximum continuous discharge current of about 1.5 A.

An alternative power source is compressed gas (CO_2) stored in a metal cylinder that provides a compact source of energy but cannot be used in aircraft travel. Also hydraulic systems offer large forces but may have leaky components.

1.6 Prosthetic socket

An important component of any upper extremity prosthesis is the method of connecting the hand to the person. For someone with a transradial amputation (an amputation through the forearm and below the elbow), a plastic socket is custom-made to fit around the tissues forming the residual limb. The manufacture of the socket is a highly skilled process that involves making a cast of the residual limb and from this an outer shell to mechanically attach the hand to the amputee. An inner lining provides comfort and suction to ensure a comfortable and secure attachment to the body. There are a range of different materials and techniques to customise the fitment to the residual limb. Further manufacturing challenges occur for the socket made for a transhumeral amputation (above the elbow) that includes an artificial elbow. Webbing straps, located posteriorly and anteriorly around the shoulders, hold and locate the socket, artificial arm and hand to the body.

Within the socket are typically sets of electrodes to detect EMG signals from residual muscles. Positioning of these electrodes requires tests to locate positions on the skin surface so that a strong and repeatable EMG signal can be produced by the amputee. Again considerable skill and experience is needed to achieve a good result. Also, the tissues under the socket are compliant, whereas the electrodes and outer socket casing are ridged, which can lead to intermittent and the occasional poor signal generation resulting in poor control of the hand [14, 15].

The power source, i.e., the batteries can also be located in the socket and may appear as a small bulge on the exterior of the outer casing.

1.7 Signals

Information gathered from the EMG electrodes and amplifiers will need to be processed into a digital form that the controller can act upon. An analogue signal from an amplifier is an AC signal that can be sampled and simply rectified and smoothed digitally by the processor in the controller. As we shall see in a later chapter, there are more sophisticated processing techniques that can be used.

1.8 Expectation

A natural hand is not able to pick up a cone from its apex using the first and second fingers opposing the thumb in a tripod grip if the opening angle at the apex is too large. Figure 1.27 shows three cones where it is impossible to pick up the cone shown in the centre of the photograph. An artificial hand has similar difficulties and should not be expected to have superhuman attributes. A journalist once asked if an artificial hand could play a piano. At a basic level a fingertip can strike a key to make one note, and so a tune with single notes can be formed but movements that require abduction or adduction of the fingers would require a difficult coordination of inputs to a controller.

1.9 Prototype hands developed at the University of Southampton

Several hands and arms have been developed at Southampton and associated controllers, sensors and algorithms [16–29]. In Figure 1.28 is a small hand design

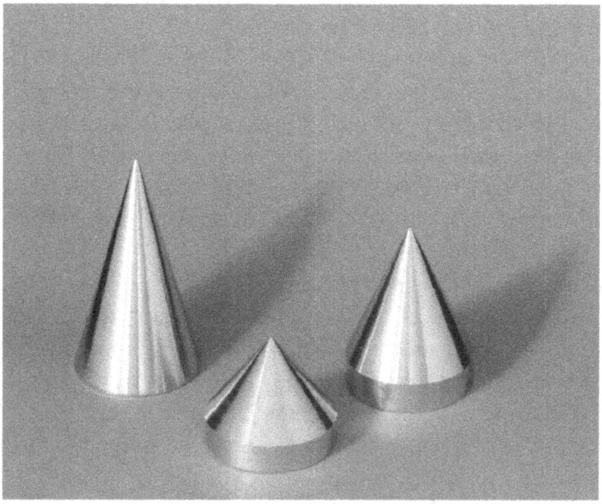

Figure 1.27 Three aluminium cones with different opening angles

that was made out of plastic material and has a mass of about 120 g with three motors, driving the first two fingers as a pair and the third and fourth fingers as a pair with one motor actuating the thumb. Other prototype hands are shown in Figures 1.29 to 1.34.

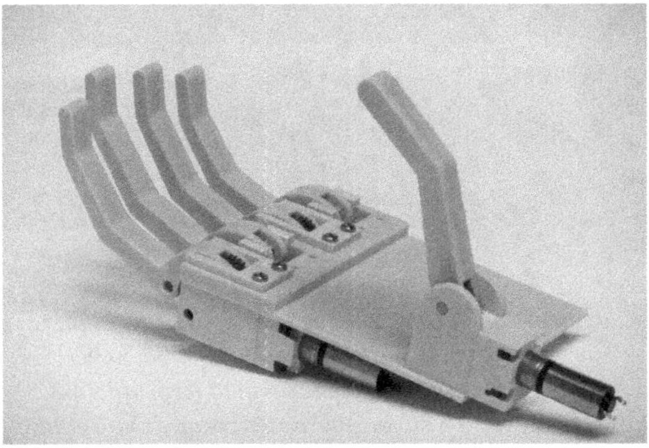

Figure 1.28 Hand designed for a child aged 5 years. It was made from polyurethane plastic (Tufset) that has a density of 1.2 g·cm^{-3}. The mass of the hand is 55 g, while the three motor drives have a mass of 65 g

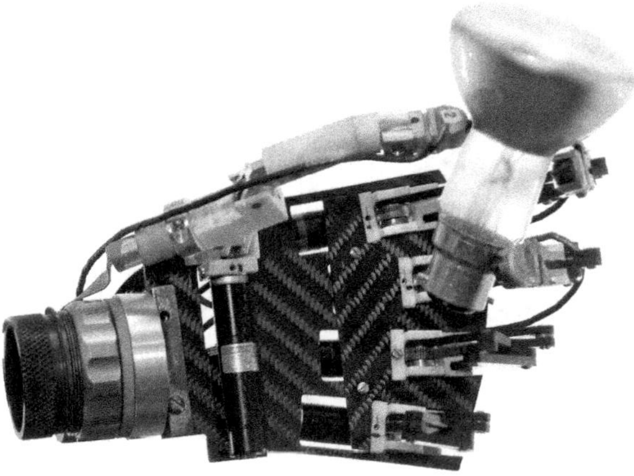

Figure 1.29 The Southampton-Remedi hand made from carbon fibre sheet holding a light bulb where the thumb is opposing the tips of the first and second fingers [13]. This design has six DC motors allowing for individual movement of the fingers

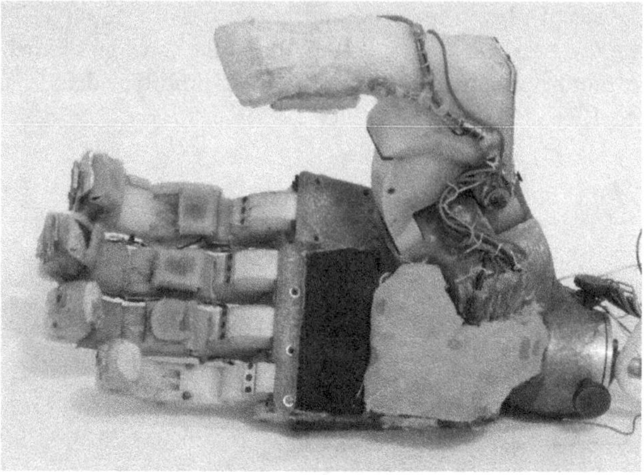

Figure 1.30 *Palmar view of a hand showing the curling fingers [25]. There are touch sensors on the palm and on the surface of the fingers. A potentiometer can be seen at the base of the thumb to measure joint angle. Force is transmitted from a motor/gearbox/capstan drive by pulling on the nylon tapes located at the first joints (metacarpophalangeal) of the fingers. The fingers curl naturally into the hand palm. The thumb has two degrees of freedom that allows it to rotate and flex. Plastic materials are used to form the finger and thumb components parts*

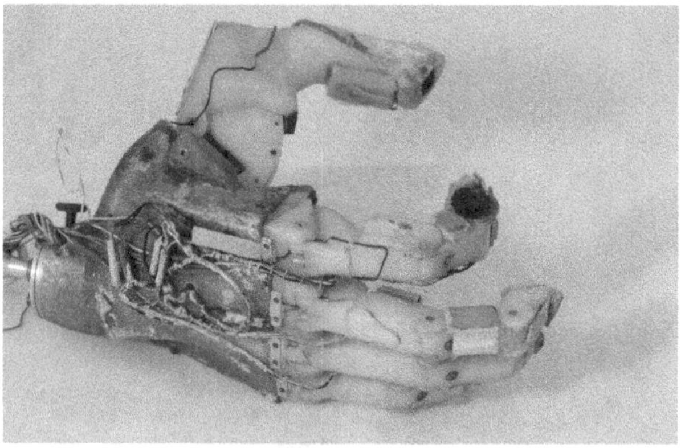

Figure 1.31 *Dorsal view of the hand with curling fingers [25]. As the fingers flex into the palm, energy is stored in elastic strips that were located along the back of the fingers but are not shown in the photograph. The white nylon cords that transmit force from the motor capstans can be seen at the joints. Pads on the side of the first finger and thumb are prototype touch and slip sensors*

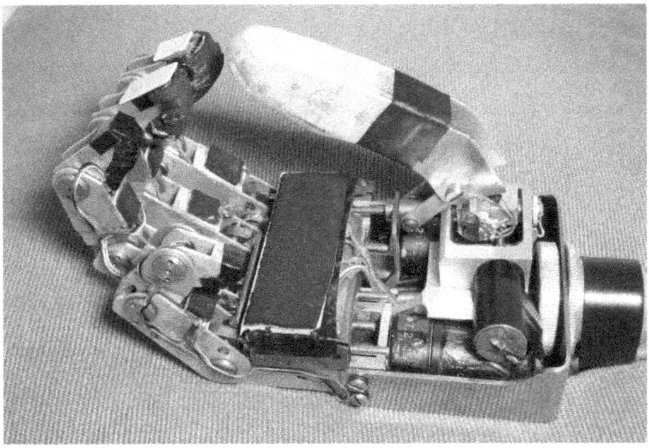

Figure 1.32 *Palmar view of a hand with a lead screw mechanism [23]. There are two motors/drives powering the fingers. One actuates the first finger, while a second motor powers the other three fingers as a group with a whiffletree mechanism allowing for differential movement between the three fingers. This mechanical design causes the curling of the fingers to be distributed around an irregular shaped object. A lead screw mechanism attached to the output shaft of the motor gearbox, pulls links curls a finger into the palm. The linking mechanism has a low mechanical advantage especially when a finger is fully extended and is straight. A motor and gearbox across the back of the palm rotates the thumb. Underneath the thumb aluminium block is a motor and gearbox to flex and extend the thumb. A potentiometer can be seen at the base of the thumb joint that is used for position feedback. Prototype sensors are located at the fingertips, thumb tip, across the links and there is a touch sensor with a large surface area located in the palm*

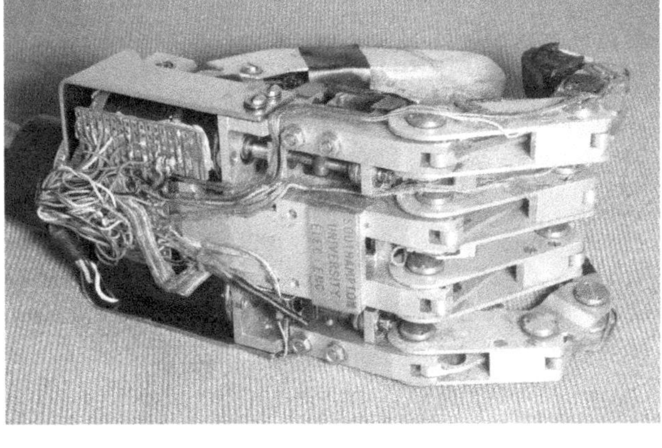

Figure 1.33 *Dorsal view a hand with a lead screw mechanism that can be seen connected to the first finger at the top of the photograph with a second lead screw driving the other three fingers at the bottom [23]*

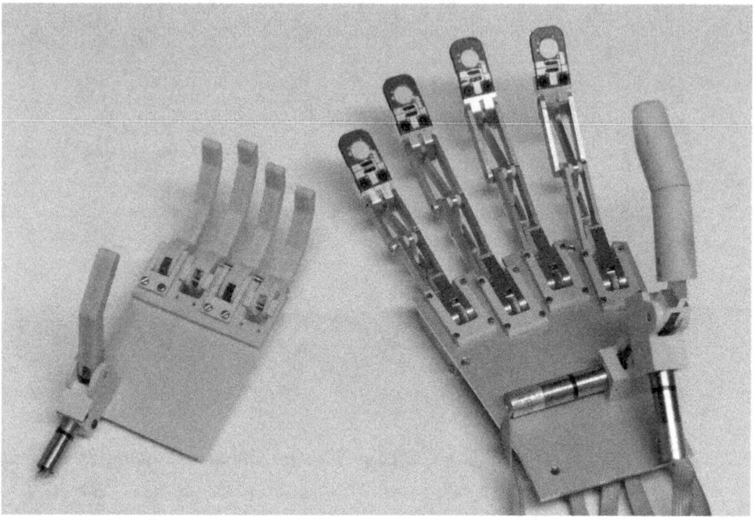

Figure 1.34 *An adult hand shown on the right [30, 31] with the hand designed for a child on the left. It has six motors and gearboxes with sensors for force, slip, texture and temperature mounted on the fingertips. The hand is made from aluminium alloys and polymers. The position of each finger and thumb are sensed by opto-electronic encoders integrated into the ends of the motors*

Table 1.1 *Organisations*

Industry

Advanced Arm Dynamics, 123 West Torrance Blvd., Suite 203, Redondo Beach, California 90277, USA
Dorset Orthopaedic Company Ltd., Unit 11, Headlands Business Park, Salisbury Road, Ringwood, Hampshire, BH24 3PB, UK
Hanger, Inc., 10910 Domain Drive, Suite 300, Austin, Texas 78758, USA
Motion Control Inc., 115 N. Wright Brothers Drive, Salt Lake City, Utah 84116, USA
Ottobock, Max-Nader-Strasse, D-37115, Duderstadt Germany
Steeper, Manufacturing Centre, Unit 7, Hunslet Trading Estate, Severn Road, Leeds, LS10 1BL, UK
Touch Bionics Inc., Unit 3 Ashwood Court, Oakbank Park Way, Livingston, EH53 0TH UK
Vincent Systems GmbH, Briet Strasse 155, 76135 Karlsruhe, Germany

Charity

Amputee Coalition of America™, Manassas, Virginia, USA
The National Trust, PO Box 574, Manvers, Rotherham, S63 3FH, UK
Wellcome Trust, Gibbs Building, 215 Euston Road, London NW1 2BE

Table 1.1 (*Continued*)

Universities
Advanced Robotics Technology and Systems, ARTS Lab, Scuola Superiore Sant'Anna, Viale le Rinaldo Piaggio 34, 56025 (Pisa) Pontedera, Italy
Biomechanical Engineering, Faculty of Mechanical Engineering, Delft University of Technology, Mekelweg 2, 2628 CD Delft, The Netherlands
Bloorview Reseach Institute, Rehabilitation Hospital, 150 Kilgour Road, Toronto, Ontario, M4G 1R8, Canada
College of Health and Social Care, University of Salford, Allerton Building, Frederick Road Campus, Salford, M6 6PU, UK
Institute of Biomaterials & Biomedical Engineering (IBBME), Rosebrugh Building, RN 407, 164 College Street, Toronto, Ontario, M5S 3G9, Canada
Institute of Biomedical Engineering, University of New Brunswick, 25 Dineen Drive, PO Box 4400, Fredericton, NB, E3B 5A3, Canada
The Johns Hopkins University Applied Physics Laboratory, 11100 Johns Hopkins Road, Laurel, Maryland 20723, USA

1.10 Sources of information

Industries, charitable organisations and universities have published documents and have websites that contain a wealth of information about artificial hands (Table 1.1). Several industries have been in existence for a long time, e.g., Otto-bock was founded in 1919. Other industries have been formed more recently to exploit advances in materials research such as Livingskin^{TM} (see Touch Bionics Inc.). Some charities have both artefacts and literature of the history of artificial hands, e.g., The Wellcome Trust.

1.11 Summary

Progress in the mechanical design, control and sensing for replacement artificial limbs has seen peaks in activity as the casualties of war return home from international conflicts. Simple mechanisms with open-loop control provide some gripping of objects. To form multiple grip patterns requires the addition of more actuators and the inclusion of sensors and closed-loop controllers. A major constraint is the mass of a hand as it is attached to the user's stump, and if it is too heavy, it will not be acceptable to a user.

References

1. Dorrance D. W. 'Artificial hand' *US patent* 1,042,413, 1912
2. Ferris J. & E. *From the surgical to the mechanical art. A treatise on the manufacture of artificial limbs*, King's Cross, W.C., London: W. & J. Balls, 1892

3. Ferris J. & E. *Manufacturers of artificial limbs & surgical appliances*, New Oxford Street, W.C., London
4. John Bell & Croyden. *Surgical appliances*, Westminster, London
5. W. R. Grossmith Ltd. *Artificial limbs, eyes, crutches, foot supplies, boots, and other appliances*, Westminster, London
6. Hugh Steeper Ltd. *Makers of artificial arms and appliances, Makers of artificial arms*, Queen Marys (Roehampton) Hospital for the Limbless, Roehampton, London
7. Kuniholm J. 'Open arms', *IEEE Spectrum*, 2009;**46**(3):36–41
8. Delaruelle L. and Sendrail M. *Textes choisis de Ambroise Paré*, vol. 31, Paris: Les textes Français; 1953
9. Lyons A. S. and Petrucelli II R. J. *Medicine an illustrated history*, New York: H. N. Abrams; 1987
10. The new encyclopaedia Britannica. In: *Micropaedia ready reference*, 9th ed., vol. 9, Chicago: Encyclopaedia Britannica; 2002, p. 736
11. Childress D. S. 'Historical aspects of powered limb prostheses', *Clinical Prosthetics & Orthotics*, 1985;**9**(1):2–13
12. Reiter R. 'Eine neue Elektrokunsthand. Grenzgebiete der Medizin', 1948; **1**(4):133–135
13. Light C. M. *An Intelligent Hand Prosthesis and Evaluation of Pathological and Prosthetic Hand Function*, PhD thesis, University of Southampton, 2000
14. Head J. S. *The Effect of Socket Movement and Electrode Contact on Myoelectric Prosthesis Control During Daily Living Activities*, PhD thesis, University of Salford, 2014
15. Head J. S., Howard D., Hutchins S. W., Kenney L., Heath G. H., and Aksenov A. Y. 'The use of an adjustable electrode housing unit to compare electrode alignment and contact variation with myoelectric prosthesis functionality: a pilot study', *Prosthetics and Orthotics International*, 2015; DOI: 10.1177/0309364614545417
16. Ahmad S. A. *Moving Approximate Entropy and Its Application to the Electromyographic Control of an Artificial Hand*, PhD thesis, University of Southampton, 2009
17. Barkhordar M. *Control of a Multifunctional Hand Prosthesis*, PhD thesis, University of Southampton, 1989
18. Baits J. C. *Basic Problems in Artificial Prehension*, PhD thesis, University of Leicester, 1970
19. Brown D. J. *The Design of an Externally-Powered Prosthetic Arm*, PhD thesis, University of Southampton, 1983
20. Codd R. D. *Development and Evaluation of Adaptive Control for a Hand Prosthesis*, PhD thesis, University of Southampton, 1976
21. Cotton D. P. J. *Thick Filmed Piezoelectric Slip Sensors for a Prosthetic Hand*, PhD thesis, University of Southampton, 2007
22. Kyberd P. J. *Digital Filter Circuits*, MSc thesis, University of Southampton, 1985

23. Kyberd P. J. *Algorithmic Control of a Multifunction Hand Prosthesis*, PhD thesis, University of Southampton, 1990
24. Light C. M. *An Intelligent Hand Prosthesis and Evaluation of Pathological and Prosthetic Hand Function*, PhD thesis, University of Southampton, 2000
25. Moore D. *Development of a Multifunctional Adaptive Hand Prosthesis,* PhD thesis, University of Southampton, 1981
26. Storey N. *Control of an Arm Prosthesis*, PhD thesis, University of Southampton, 1978
27. Swain I. D. *Adaptive Control of an Arm Prosthesis*, PhD thesis, University of Southampton, 1982
28. Todd R. W. *Adaptive Control of a Hand Prosthesis*, PhD thesis, University of Southampton, 1971
29. Redman T. R. *The Design of a Myoelectrically Controlled Hand with Multiple Actuators for Children*, PhD thesis, University of Southampton, 2016
30. Cranny A., Cotton D. P. J., Chappell P. H., Beeby S. P., and White N. M. 'Thick-film force and slip sensors for a prosthetic hand', *Sensors Actuat A: Phys*, 2005;**123–124**:162–171
31. Cranny A., Cotton D. P. J., Chappell P. H., Beeby S. P., and White N. M. 'Thick-film force and slip sensors for a prosthetic hand', *Measurement Science and Technology*, 2005;**16**:931–941

Bibliography

Muzumdar A., ed. *Powered Upper Limb Prostheses* (Springer-Verlag, Berlin, Heidelberg, ISBN: 978-3-642-62302-8, 2004)

Castelli V. P. and Troncossi M., eds. *Grasping the Future: Advances in Powered Upper Limb Prosthetics* (Bentham Science, ISBN: 978-1-60805-438-1, 2012)

Merletti R. *Electromyography: physiology, engineering, and noninvasive applications* (Piscataway, NJ: IEEE Press; Hoboken, NJ: Wiley-Interscience, ISBN 978-0-471675808, 2004)

Basmajian J. V. *Muscles alive: their functions revealed by electromyography* (2nd ed., Baltimore: Williams & Wilkins, 1967)

Dorf R. C. *Modern control systems* (Pearson, Harlow, 12th ed, ISBN: 978-1-292024059, 2103)

Hall J. G., Allanson J. E., Gripp K. W., and Slavotinek A. M. *Handbook of physical measurements* (Oxford University Press, Oxford, New York, ISBN 9780195301496, 2006)

Illis L. S., ed. *Neurological rehabilitation*, Blackwell Scientific Publications, Oxford, , ISBN 0-632-03282-0

Kapandji I. A. *The physiology of the joints annotated diagrams of the mechanics of the human joints. Volume 1: The upper limb* (Churchill Livingstone, Edinburgh, London, Melbourne and New York, 5th ed., ISBN 0 443 02504 5, 1982)

Chapter 2

Mechanisms

A passive artificial hand that has no power source or control over its movement can be made from a range of materials whose physical properties are important to provide a lifelike visual impact, feel and durability. In contrast, a hand that needs to be designed to hold and manipulate objects requires as at least some form of mechanical structure, c.f., a skeleton but also other components so that it is functional. It has a palm or central structure for the attachment of finger joints and links that is similar to the anatomy of a natural hand (Figure 2.1). Also there is provision for actuators, i.e., electric motors or if the device is body powered, cables to react against the mechanism.

For a powered anthropomorphic hand, choices are made about which of the fingers and thumb should be powered. A single actuator could move the first finger or groups of fingers and the thumb to form pinch grips where the fingertips oppose the thumb tip. With two actuators a finger or group of fingers can move independently of the powered thumb. Alternatively, one actuator could move both the first finger and thumb together and the second actuator moves the other fingers. Three actuators allow for the thumb to have two degrees of freedom with the third actuator powering all the fingers. Alternatively, the first finger could be powered with one actuator and the three other fingers with a second actuator. The powered thumb then has only one movement of extension/flexion and no rotation. The thumb can also have no power and be moved into position using a natural hand, in which case all three actuators are available for moving the fingers. With four actuators, there are more possible combinations for grip patterns but each additional actuator adds mass not only to the hand but also is in need of more coordination and algorithmic control of the fingers and thumb.

2.1 Materials

The physical properties of the materials used in the manufacture an artificial hand need careful scrutiny. The most important physical property is the density of the material since the mass of a hand must be kept as low as possible. In the selection of a candidate material for a particular part, often a good material can be found that has a low density but is weak and so has to be rejected. Table 2.1 shows some of the important properties of materials. In general, there are metals, metal alloys, plastics, polymers and composite materials.

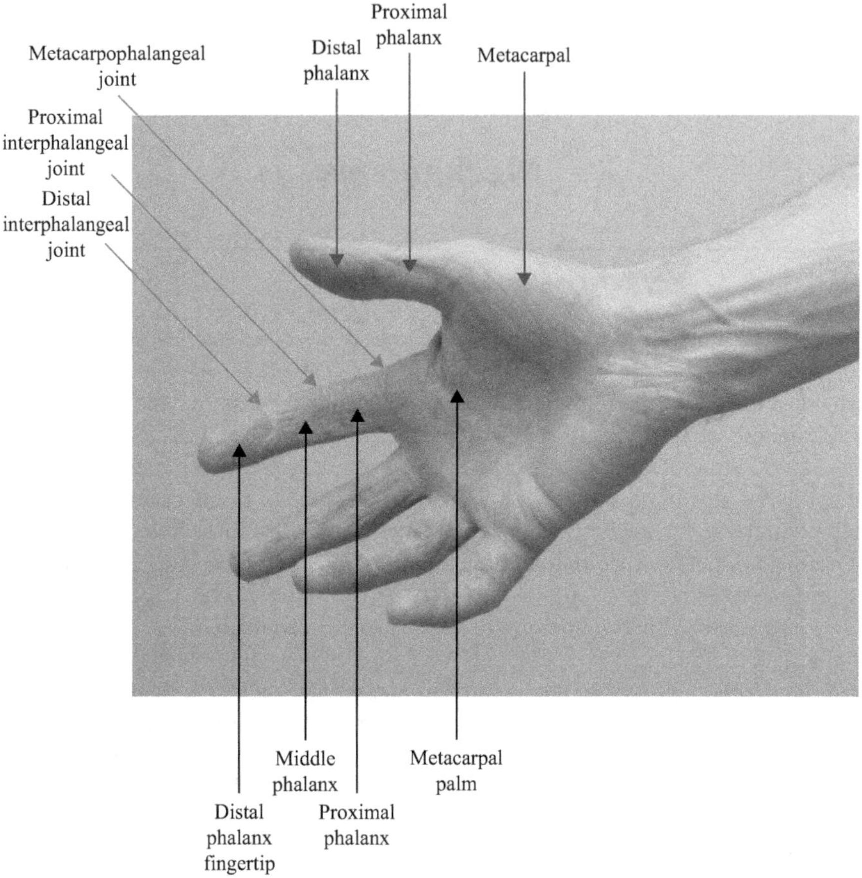

Figure 2.1 Diagram showing positions of the bones of the first finger and thumb with the joints of the first finger. These are the metacarpal, proximal phalanx, middle phalanx and distal phalanx with the metacarpophalangeal joint, proximal interphalangeal joint and distal interphalangeal joint

Table 2.1 Material characteristics

Light-weight low density	Strong high tensile strength	Easily machined	Bio-medically compatible	Good corrosion resistance	Low cost	High hardness/ impact strength

Aluminium alloys rather than pure aluminium are good materials for the structural parts of an artificial hand. They have a low density compared to other metal alloys such as steel and have a range of good physical properties. The alloy 7075, e.g., has high strength and hardness and is good to machine but has limited

Table 2.2 Metals

Material	Tensile modulus, GPa	Tensile strength, MPa	Melting point, °C	Density, g·cm^{-3}	Electrical resistivity, μΩcm	Hardness
Aluminium alloy	70	200–500	450–630	2.8	5.2	60–150
Brass	100	300	900	8.5	6.4	80
Stainless steel	200	700	1400	8.0	70	60
Titanium	120	340	1660	4.5	54	60

Table 2.3 Plastics polymers and composites

Material	Tensile modulus, GPa	Tensile strength, MPa	Working temperature, °C	Density, g·cm^{-3}	Electrical resistivity, Ωcm	Hardness	Coefficient of friction
Carbon-epoxy	70	90		1.6			
Polycarbonate	6	70	140	1.4	10^{16}		
Polymethyl-methacrylate (Acrylic)	2.9	80	160	1.2	10^{16}	95	
Polypropylene	1.2	30	110	0.9	10^{17}		0.2
Polytetra-fluoroethylene	0.5	25	220	2.2	10^{18}	50	0.1
polyimide	2.5	110	290	1.4	10^{18}	80	0.42

resistance to corrosion. It is used widely in the aerospace industries. The alloy 5251 has a medium strength with a high resistance to corrosion and is good to machine. Table 2.2 illustrates the high strength and melting points of metals and their alloys. They are useful for places where there are high stresses such as the shafts joining finger links together.

There are a wide range of suitable plastic, polymer and composite materials that have low densities compared to metals and their alloys (Table 2.3).

2.2 Simple clamps

In its simplest form in Figure 2.2, an artificial hand has a palm or base and a finger (or thumb). The force produced at the fingertip or reaction force on the object, f_R is

$$f_R = \frac{T}{l_f} \tag{2.1}$$

where T is the torque applied to the finger shaft by an actuator and l_f is the finger length. Clockwise rotation of the finger opens the hand and accommodates an object whose size depends on the finger geometry and maximum angle, θ.

The base can be a flat palm with an opposing finger. As the finger is rigid, it can be curved and shaped into a more natural appearance than the simple

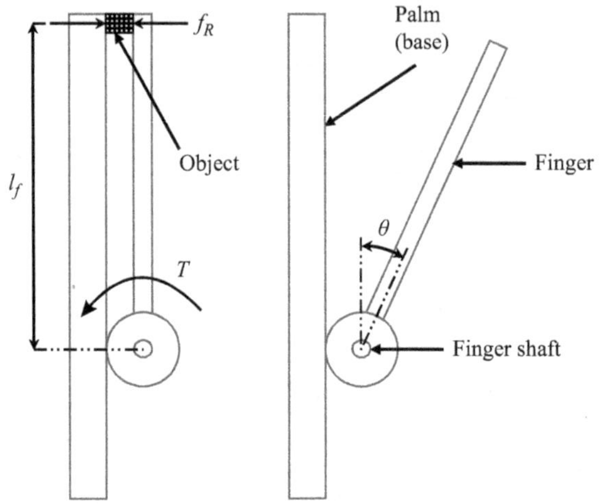

Figure 2.2 Diagrammatic side view of a simple artificial hand

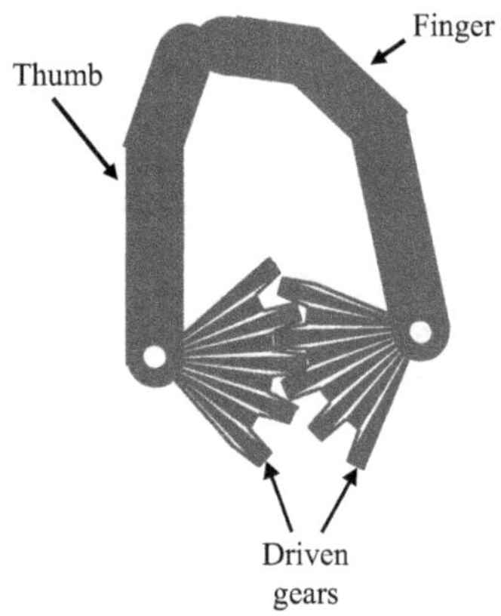

Figure 2.3 Tradition arrangement of a single degree of freedom hand showing the coupled finger(s) and thumb

rectangular block shown in Figure 2.2. For many decades, the traditional design is a finger (or the first and second fingers together forming a tripod grip) and thumb driven by a single actuator through a set of gears (Figures 2.3 and 2.4).

A single motor and gearbox drives either the finger or thumb. The simple design is robust. It has a safety mechanism, using a preloaded spring so that the fingers and thumb can be forced to break them apart. Unpowered fingers (the third and fourth) are coupled to the other two fingers by compliant materials and the cosmesis (glove). This type of hand is usually designed for a tip (pinch grip) or tripod grip using finger and thumb tips, but this hand is also very good at holding spherical objects.

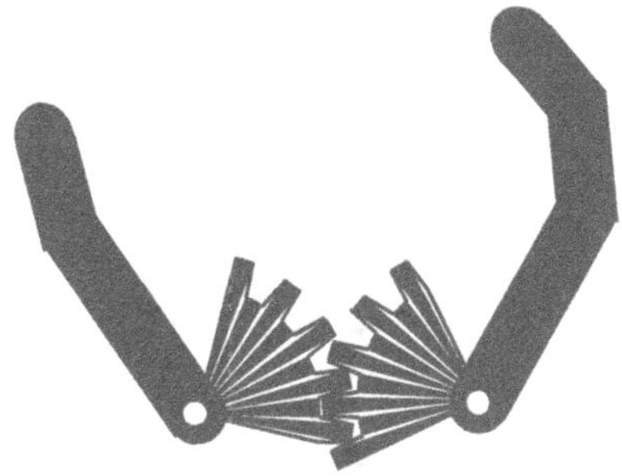

Figure 2.4 Traditional hand opened by driving the gears

2.3 Natural curling fingers

In a human, skeletal muscles are contracted and pull on tendons connected to bony structures that change position to apply force during gripping. A pair of muscles acts together; one muscle pulls a structure in one direction, while a second muscle (the antagonist) pulls the structure in the opposite direction. The extensor digitorum muscle extends the fingers (and wrist) as it is located in the dorsal side of the forearm, and tendons are attached to the dorsal sides of the distal phalanges (bones of the fingertips). The flexor digitorum superficialis muscle is also located in the forearm, and tendons are attached to the palmar sides of the middle phalanges. Contraction of this muscle causes the fingers to flex first at the middle phalanges and then at the fingertips. By contracting the extensor muscle the hand is opened, and on contraction of the flexor muscle the hand can close round an object. In order to produce a force and react against a bony structure, the other end of the extensor digitorum muscle is attached to the coronoid process of the ulna, the medial epicondyle of the humerus and the anterior upper surface of the radius. The flexor digitorum superficialis muscle is attached in the same place as the extensor muscle.

The same principle can be applied in an artificial hand through the use of actuators and cords. A single DC motor and gearbox with a capstan is shown in Figures 2.5 and 2.6. The finger is extended away from the palm as the capstan is rotated anticlockwise against the spring tension. Decreasing the power to the motor flexes the finger into the palm under the release of energy from the spring. There are several different designs for this mechanism. Rather than attaching the cord to the spring and relying on friction between the finger pulley and cord, it can be returned back to the capstan but this arrangement requires some pre-tensioning of the cord with a spring, otherwise there will be some slack in the drive mechanism. However, the mechanism allows for active griping by reversing the polarity of the voltage applied to the motor. When there is no power in the motor the finger can be backdriven causing an object held in the hand to be released. This lack of grip, with no power, can be overcome with the application of a mechanical brake. Either an electromechanical brake or a ratchet and pawl with an electrical release can be used. A controller will need to coordinate the release and application of the brake with supplying power to the motor. A controller can achieve a smooth transition

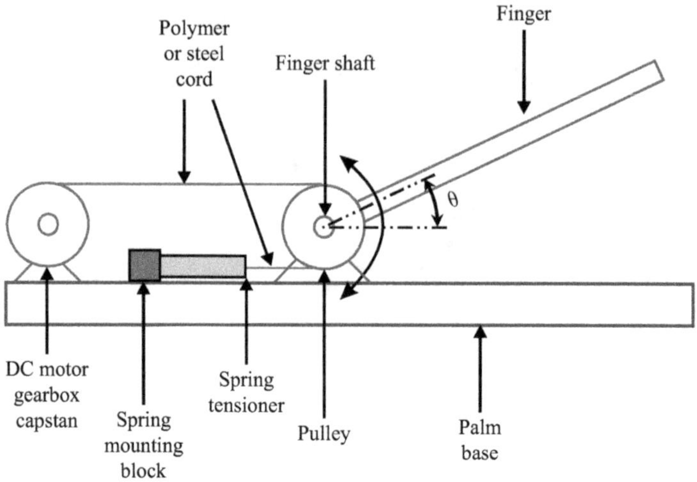

Figure 2.5 Diagrammatic side view of a motor, gearbox and pulley with a spring tensioner

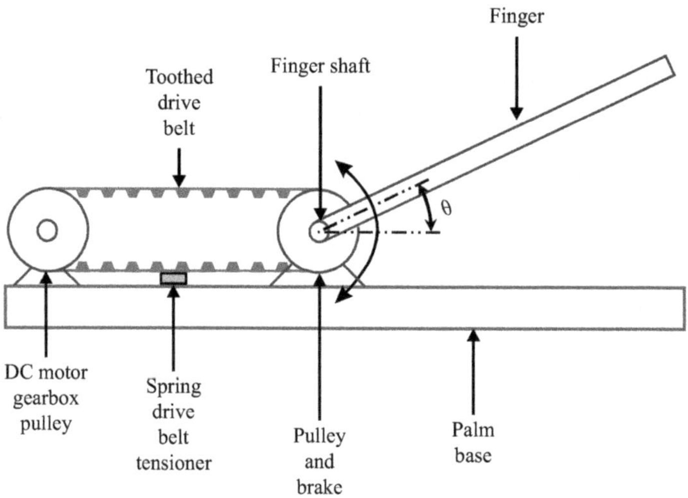

Figure 2.6 Diagrammatic side view of a mechanism with a motor, gearbox, pulley, toothed drive belt and spring tensioner

between active power from the motor and a constant grip from the brake depending on the time constants of the devices.

2.4 Curling fingers and pulleys

The static appearance of a simple hand can show the curl of a finger or thumb but its single pivot point does not allow for anthropomorphic movement. A more realistic curling action can be achieved with the mechanism shown in Figure 2.7.

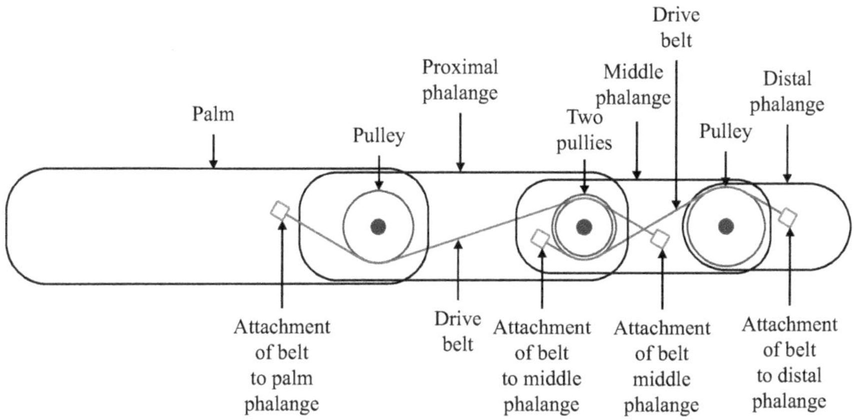

Figure 2.7 Diagrammatic side view of a curling finger with three joints

One of the disadvantages of this design is that the grip force generated can be low due to the mechanical disadvantage produced by the links especially when a finger is straight.

Moore studied the design of a finger that has a natural curling action requiring joints [1]. The example, shown in Figure 2.7, has a palm and three parts to the finger representing the proximal, middle and distal phalanges. Two drive belts constrain the curling action of the finger. A motor and gearbox, mounted transversely in the palm, rotate the proximal phalange. The distal end of the proximal phalange is raised causing tension to be developed in the drive belt connecting the palm to the middle phalange. The belt curls round the pulley at the axis of the palm and proximal phalange and also the pulley on the axle between the proximal and middle phalanges. The angle, between the axis of the proximal and middle phalanges, decreases from 180 degrees. Similarly, a second drive belt connecting the middle phalange to the distal phalange reduces the angle made between the middle and distal phalanges. Shown in Figure 2.8 are the links in various positions as the proximal phalange is rotated through 90 degrees. The positions of the joints and fingertip are shown in Figure 2.9.

The trajectory of the fingertip and joints can be designed by adjusting the radii of the pulleys and the lengths of the phalanges. The plots shown in the figures are with the dimensions given in Table 2.4.

Tensions are developed in the two belts and are related to the force at the fingertip that is normal to the distal phalange. With reference to Figure 2.10, taking moments about the axis of the proximal joint

$$T_p = F_p r_p \tag{2.2}$$

where T_p is the input torque produced from the output of the gearbox, F_p is the tension in the drive belt between the palm and distal phalange and r_p is the radius of the proximal pulley.

For the middle joint,

$$T = F_p r_{m1} \tag{2.3}$$

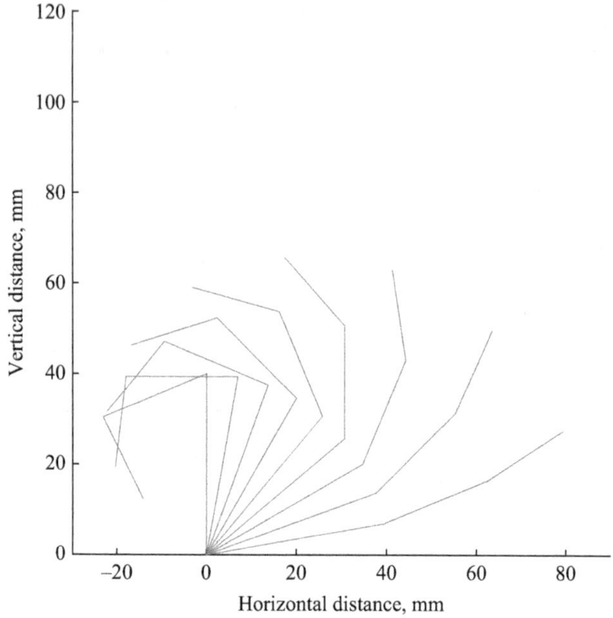

Figure 2.8 *Diagrammatic side view showing the location of the phalanges as the proximal phalange is rotated 90 degrees in 10-degree steps. The origin is the centre of the joint connecting the proximal phalange to the distal phalange*

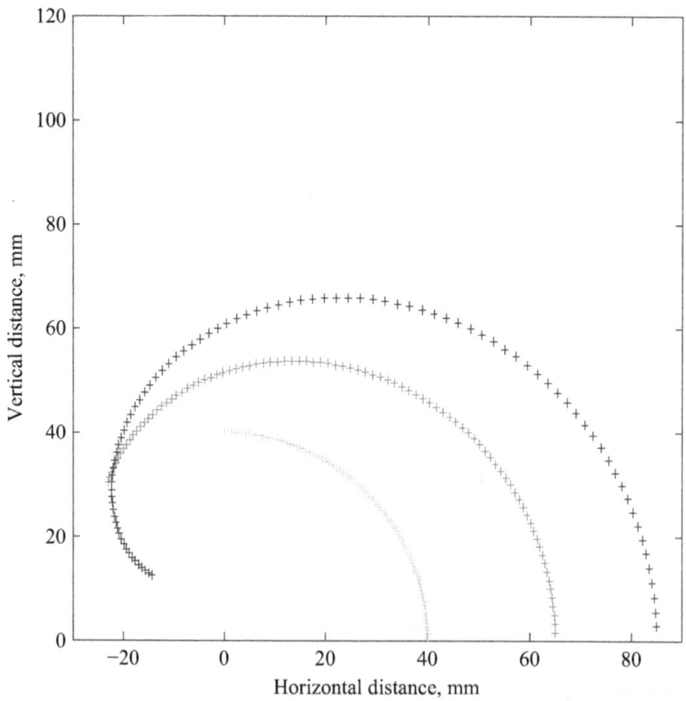

Figure 2.9 *Positions of the end of the phalanges as the proximal phalange is rotated through 90 degrees in 1-degree steps*

Table 2.4 Dimensions of the finger components. All the dimensions are in millimetres

Pulley		**Radius**	**Phalange**		**Length**
Proximal	r_p	5	Proximal	l_p	40
Input middle	r_{m1}	4	Middle	l_m	25
Output middle	r_{m2}	5	Distal	l_d	20
Distal	r_d	6			

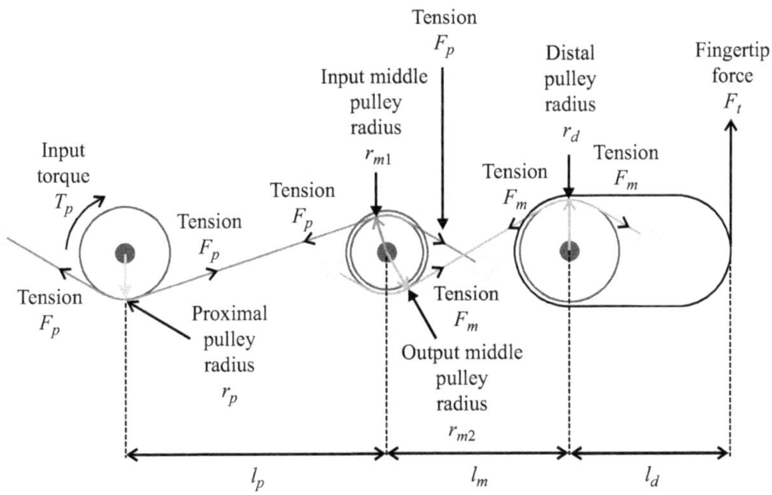

Figure 2.10 Diagrammatic side view of the pulley and tendon mechanism

where F_m is the tension in the drive belt between the middle and distal phalanges and r_{m1} is the radius of the input middle pulley.

At the middle joint,

$$T = F_m r_{m2} \tag{2.4}$$

where r_{m2} is the radius of the output middle pulley r_d is the radius of the distal pulley.

At the distal phalange,

$$F_m r_d = F_t l_d \tag{2.5}$$

where F_t is the force normal to the distal phalange and l_d is the length of the distal phalange.

Combining these equations and eliminating F_m and F_p

$$F_t = \frac{T_p}{r_p}\frac{r_{m1}}{r_{m2}}\frac{r_d}{l_d} \tag{2.6}$$

2.5 Curling fingers and one four-bar linkage

Rotation of a link about a point with another link crossing it results in a mechanism that curls the finger joints in a natural manner. In Figure 2.11, on the left is the palm, where O is the metacarpophalangeal joint and on the right are the middle distal and phalanges. The links OB and AC form the proximal phalange. Rotation of the link OB in a counterclockwise sense moves the links upwards and curls the finger (Figure 2.12). The fingertip trajectory has a natural curl into the palm (Figure 2.13).

A prototype mechanism is shown in Figure 2.14, which was assembled to test the movement of the parts and to demonstrate the principle operation of the links. The worm and wheel are also shown where the axes of the two components are orthogonal. A small grub screw can be seen on the top of the palm block that with a

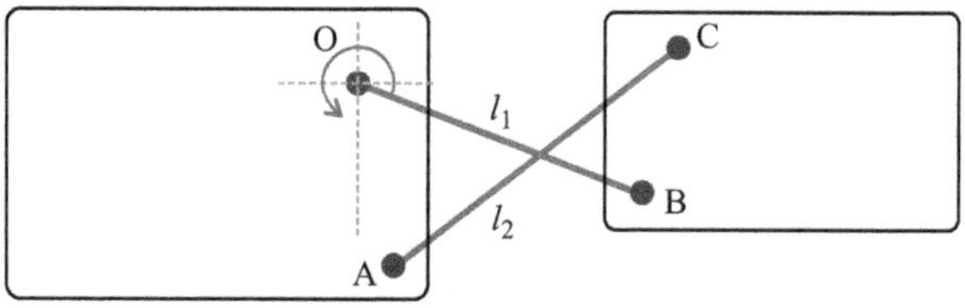

Figure 2.11 One set of crossed links

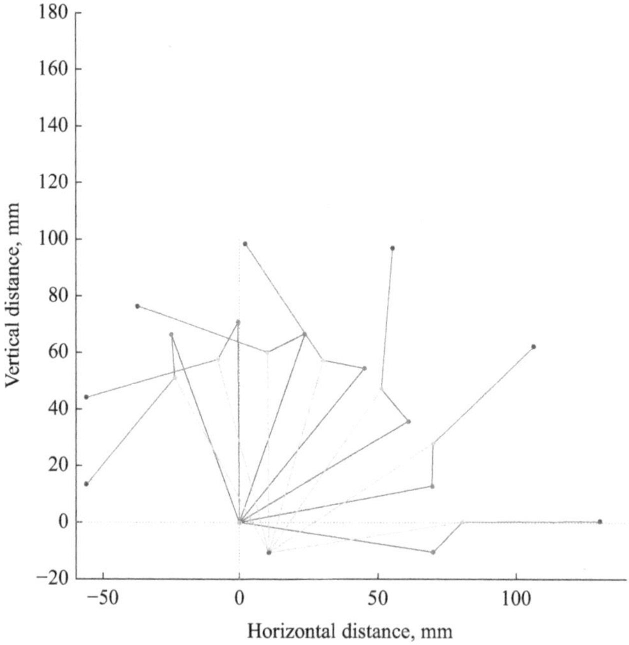

Figure 2.12 Single joint links showing trajectories every 20 degrees from 0 to 130 degrees rotation of link OB

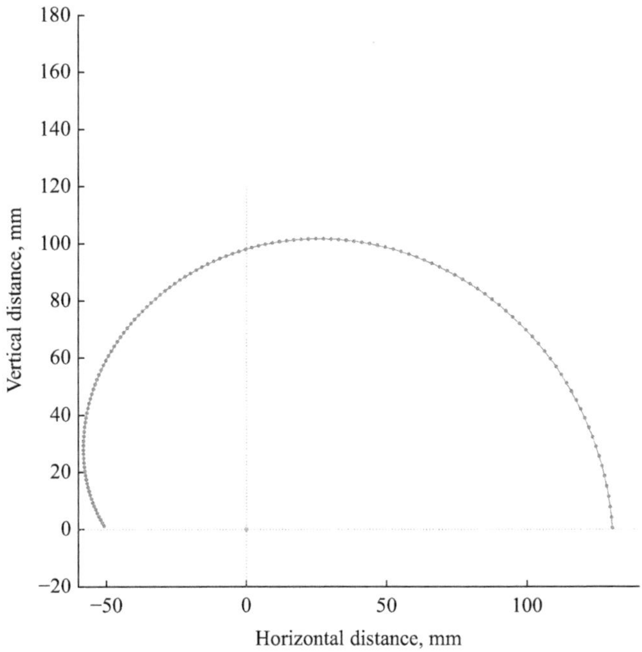

Figure 2.13 Single joint links showing trajectory of the tip every one degree from 0 to 130 degrees rotation of link OB

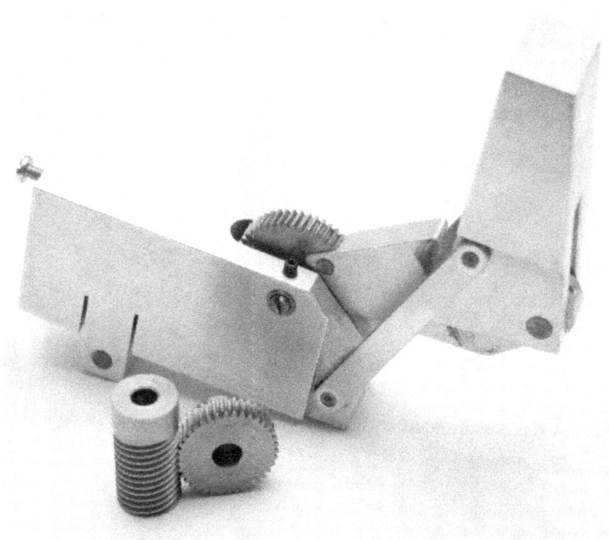

Figure 2.14 Prototype mechanism with worm and wheel

small cam, allowed for the distance between the two axes to be adjusted so that the meshing of the gears did not cause unnecessary wear and friction by being either too tight or too loose. From this initial prototype finger, a hand with a finger and thumb was made (Figure 2.15). This design is a low cost and reliable solution with the benefit of using low-density plastic materials for the gearbox housings of the worms and wheels. Two other fingers (not shown) can be added for the third and fourth fingers, which can be active or passive. The motors and gearboxes, shown in the figures, are low cost and in a practical hand would be replaced with smaller and more powerful ones. The thumb has a wide opening range (Figures 2.16 and 2.17) but does not have a curling link mechanism.

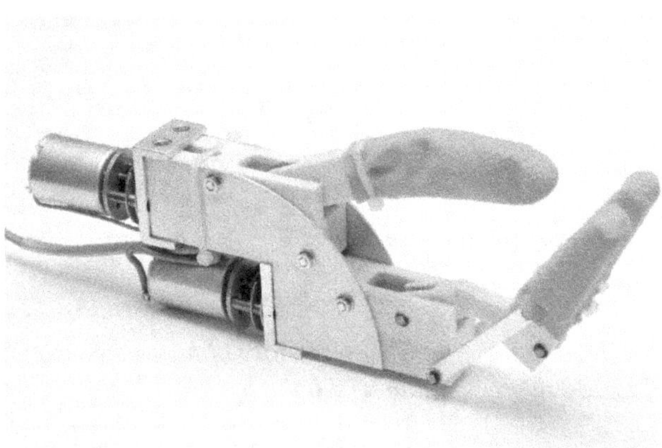

Figure 2.15 A prototype hand with a powered thumb, first and second fingers. Fingers 3 and 4 would be passively coupled to the first two fingers

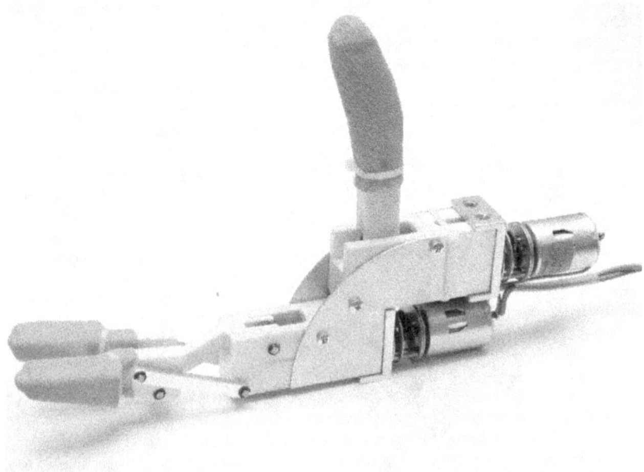

Figure 2.16 A prototype hand with the thumb fully extended

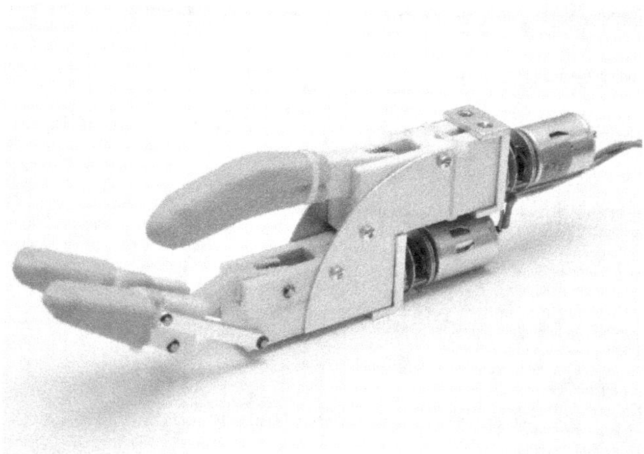

Figure 2.17 A prototype hand with the fingers fully extended and the thumb fully flexed

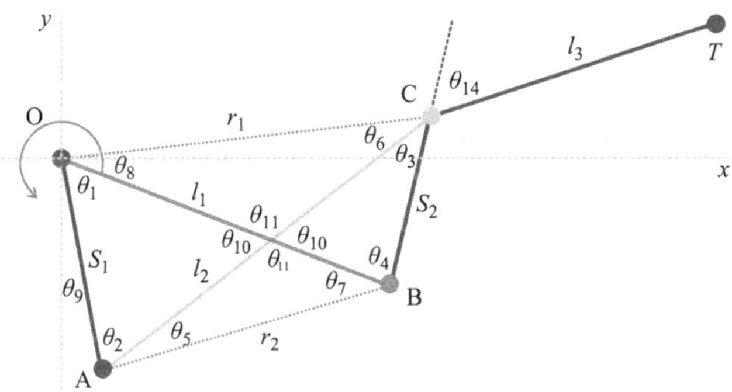

Figure 2.18 Diagram of a set of crossed links of a four-bar linkage for analysis of the mechanism

In two-dimensional space, the mechanism can be analysed in various ways by stating the problem in terms of vectors, complex numbers or trigonometry. The linkages are shown in Figure 2.18. OA, AC, CB and BO are the four links that are constant parameters in the analysis. Distances r_1 and r_2 vary as the input bar, OB is rotated in a counterclockwise direction. Using standard trigonometry, the relationship between the angle of OB with respect to the palm surface (horizontal, x-axis) and the tip, T, can be determined. The angle OB with respect to the x-axis is

$$90 - \theta_1 - \theta_9$$

Since θ_9 is fixed by the location of the joints O and A in the palm block, the fingertip can be moved by varying θ_1.

The dimension, r_2, is determined from the triangle OAB.

$$r_2 = \left(s_1^2 + l_1^2 - 2s_1 l_1 \cos\theta_1\right)^{1/2} \tag{2.7}$$

The angles in triangle OAB are θ_7 and $(\theta_2 + \theta_5)$.

$$\theta_7 = 2\cos^{-1}\left(\frac{sm_7(sm_7 - s_1)}{r_2 l_1}\right)^{1/2} \tag{2.8}$$

where

$$sm_7 = \frac{r_2 + s_1 + l_1}{2} \tag{2.9}$$

Similarly, $(\theta_2 + \theta_5)$ is determined from triangle OAB.

$$(\theta_2 + \theta_5) = 2\cos^{-1}\left(\frac{sm_{25}(sm_{25} - s_2)}{r_2 s_1}\right)^{1/2} \tag{2.10}$$

where

$$sm_{25} = \frac{r_2 + s_1 + l_1}{2} \tag{2.11}$$

Similarly, θ_5 is determined from triangle ABC.

$$\theta_5 = 2\cos^{-1}\left(\frac{sm_5(sm_5 - s_2)}{r_2 l_2}\right)^{1/2} \tag{2.12}$$

where

$$sm_5 = \frac{r_2 + s_2 + l_2}{2} \tag{2.13}$$

Then, angle θ_2 is simply

$$\theta_2 = (\theta_2 + \theta_5) - \theta_5 \tag{2.14}$$

The dimension, r_1 is determined from triangle OAC

$$r_1 = \left(s_1^2 + l_2^2 - 2s_1 l_2 \cos\theta_2\right)^{1/2} \tag{2.15}$$

The angle θ_8 is determined from triangle OBC

$$\theta_8 = 2\cos^{-1}\left(\frac{sm_8(sm_8 - s_2)}{r_1 l_1}\right)^{1/2} \tag{2.16}$$

$$sm_8 = \frac{r_1 + s_2 + l_1}{2} \tag{2.17}$$

$$\theta_{10} = 180 - \theta_1 - \theta_2 \tag{2.18}$$

From triangle ABC, θ_3 is determined.

$$\theta_3 = 2\cos^{-1}\left(\frac{sm_3(sm_3 - r_2)}{s_2 l_2}\right)^{1/2} \tag{2.19}$$

$$\theta_{11} = \frac{(360 - 2\,\theta_{10})}{2} \tag{2.20}$$

$$\theta_6 = \theta_{10} - \theta_8 \tag{2.21}$$

From triangle ABC, θ_3 is determined.

$$\theta_3 = 2\cos^{-1}\left(\frac{sm_3(sm_3 - r_2)}{s_2 l_2}\right)^{1/2} \tag{2.22}$$

$$sm_3 = \frac{r_2 + s_2 + l_2}{2} \tag{2.23}$$

The (x, y) coordinates of joints A, B and C are found with respect to the origin O by resolving them using the dimensions l_1, l_2, s_1, s_2, r_1, r_2 and the angles (note subtract 90 degrees).

Joint A

$$x_A = s_1 \cos\theta_9 \tag{2.24}$$

$$y_A = s_1 \sin\theta_9 \tag{2.25}$$

Joint B

$$x_B = l_1 \cos(\theta_1 + \theta_9) \tag{2.26}$$

$$y_B = l_1 \sin(\theta_1 + \theta_9) \tag{2.27}$$

Joint C

$$x_C = r_1 \cos(\theta_1 + \theta_8 + \theta_9) \tag{2.28}$$

$$y_C = r_1 \sin(\theta_1 + \theta_8 + \theta_9) \tag{2.29}$$

The medial and distal phalanges are one component with no distal interphalangeal joint. The link BC is at an angle, θ_{14} to the medial–distal phalanges, CT. The coordinates of the fingertip are found by determining the angle of link BC with respect to the x-axis, subtracting it from θ_{14} and adding the components to those of C as follows.

The unit components of link BC are

$$x_{uBC} = \frac{(x_C - x_B)}{s_2} \tag{2.30}$$

$$y_{uBC} = \frac{(y_C - y_B)}{s_2} \tag{2.31}$$

$$\theta_{BC} = \tan^{-1}\frac{y_{uBC}}{x_{uBC}} \tag{2.32}$$

The fingertip coordinates are

$$x_T = x_C + l_3 \cos(\theta_{BC} - \theta_{14}) \tag{2.33}$$

$$y_T = y_C + l_3 \sin(\theta_{BC} - \theta_{14}) \tag{2.34}$$

Forces are produced in the finger mechanism to hold an object by generating a counterclockwise torque at the joint O, in the link OB shown in Figure 2.18 from a worm wheel, gearbox and an electric motor assembly. At the fingertip, *T*, a force normal to the link CT can be determined from the mechanism geometry. This relationship between the input link, OB, and the output link, AC, is not linear. It is represented by the transmission ratio that is similar in action to that of a spur gear ratio except that unlike a standard gearbox where the ratio is constant as the gears rotate, in the finger mechanism the ratio varies. Rothenhofer, Walsh and Slocum have analysed different mechanisms and the transmission ratio for the input and output of four-bar mechanisms [2].

For a gearbox with an input angle, θ_i, and an output angle, θ_o the gearbox ratio, G_r, is

$$G_r = \frac{\frac{d\theta_o}{dt}}{\frac{d\theta_i}{dt}} \tag{2.35}$$

A similar angular ratio can be determined for the input and output angles of the links that defines the transmission ratio. In Figure 2.18 the angle, θ_1, increases as the link OB rotates counterclockwise while the angle, θ_2, decreases which is defining the movement of the link CB and hence CT since the component BCT is made from a single piece of material. The input torque is applied by moving link OB with respect to the link OA, so link OA is the 'base' of the mechanism. In finding the angular input–output relationship, it is the rate of change of the angle, θ_1 with respect to rate of change of the link AC that is required to find the transmission ratio, t_r. The angle of link AC with respect to link OA is $(180 - \theta_2)$.

$$t_r = \frac{\frac{d\theta_2}{dt}}{\frac{d\theta_1}{dt}} = \frac{d\theta_2}{d\theta_1} \tag{2.36}$$

Figure 2.18 is redrawn in Figure 2.19 where the link OA is horizontal. The following analysis is for the case where the two links OB and AC are of equal length and the two links OA and BC are also of equal length. In this case, there is symmetry in the mechanism where the two triangles with angles θ_1, θ_2 and θ_{10} and angles θ_3, θ_4 and θ_{10} have the same dimensions. They also have the equal angles.

$$\theta_1 = \theta_3 \tag{2.37}$$

$$\theta_2 = \theta_4 \tag{2.38}$$

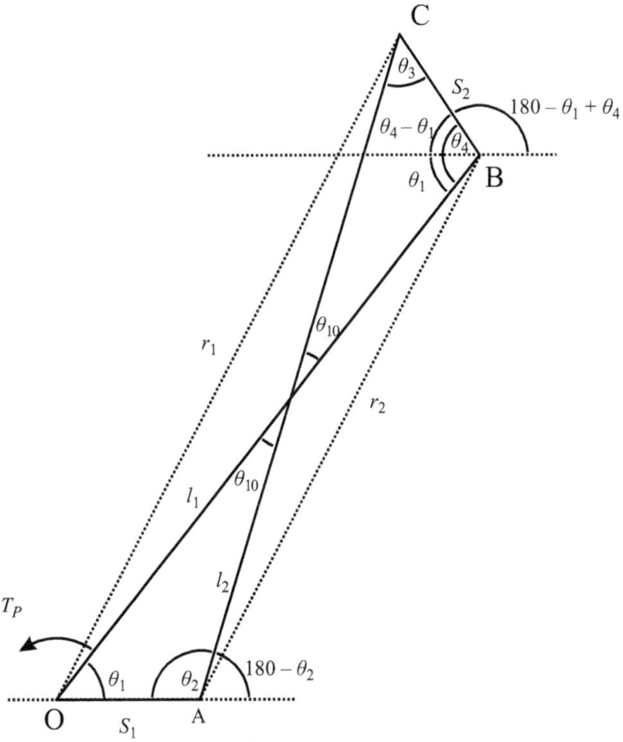

Figure 2.19 Redrawn figure of the mechanism shown in Figure 2.18 where the base is the link OA

The intersection of the links OA and BC divides the lengths l_1 *and* l_2 in proportions that are the same.

$$l_1 = l_2 = a + b \tag{2.39}$$

Applying the sine law to the two triangles and using (2.38) and (2.37)

$$\frac{a}{\sin\theta_4} = \frac{b}{\sin\theta_1} = \frac{s_1}{\sin\theta_{10}} = \frac{s_1}{\sin(180 - (\theta_1 + \theta_4))} = \frac{s_1}{\sin(\theta_1 + \theta_4)} \tag{2.40}$$

From (2.40)

$$a = \frac{b\sin\theta_4}{\sin\theta_1} \tag{2.41}$$

Substituting (2.41) into (2.39)

$$\frac{b\sin\theta_4}{\sin\theta_1} + b = l_1 \tag{2.42}$$

From (2.40)

$$b = \frac{s_1 \sin\theta_1}{\sin(\theta_1 + \theta_4)} \tag{2.43}$$

Substituting (2.43) into (2.42)

$$\frac{s_1 \sin\theta_1}{\sin(\theta_1 + \theta_4)}\left(\frac{\sin\theta_4 + \sin\theta_1}{\sin\theta_1}\right) = l_1 \tag{2.44}$$

Rearranging

$$s_1 \sin\theta_4 + s_1 \sin\theta_1 = l_1 \sin(\theta_1 + \theta_4) \tag{2.45}$$

$$s_1 \sin\theta_4 + s_1 \sin\theta_1 - l_1 \sin\theta_1 \cos\theta_4 - l_1 \cos\theta_1 \sin\theta_4 = 0 \tag{2.46}$$

$$\sin\theta_1(s_1 - l_1 \cos\theta_4) = \sin\theta_4(l_1 \cos\theta_1 - s_1) \tag{2.47}$$

$$\frac{\sin\theta_1}{(l_1 \cos\theta_1 - s_1)} = \frac{\sin\theta_4}{(s_1 - l_1 \cos\theta_4)} \tag{2.48}$$

To determine the transmission ratio, (2.46) is differentiated with respect to θ_1 to find the relationship between $\frac{d\theta_4}{d\theta_1}$ and the two angles, θ_1 and θ_4.

$$\begin{aligned} s_1 \cos\theta_4 \frac{\mathrm{d}\theta_4}{\mathrm{d}\theta_1} + s_1 \cos\theta_1 - l_1 \cos\theta_1 \cos\theta_4 - l_1 \sin\theta_1(-\sin\theta_4)\frac{\mathrm{d}\theta_4}{\mathrm{d}\theta_1} \\ - l_1(-\sin\theta_1)\sin\theta_4 - l_1 \cos\theta_1 \cos\theta_4 \frac{\mathrm{d}\theta_4}{\mathrm{d}\theta_1} = 0 \end{aligned} \tag{2.49}$$

Rearranging (2.49)

$$\begin{aligned} (s_1 \cos\theta_4 + l_1 \sin\theta_1 \sin\theta_4 - l_1 \cos\theta_1 \cos\theta_4)\frac{\mathrm{d}\theta_4}{\mathrm{d}\theta_1} + s_1 \cos\theta_1 \\ - l_1 \cos\theta_1 \cos\theta_4 + l_1 \sin\theta_1 \sin\theta_4 = 0 \end{aligned} \tag{2.50}$$

$$(s_1 \cos\theta_4 - l_1 \cos(\theta_1 + \theta_4))\frac{d\theta_4}{d\theta_1} = -s_1 \cos\theta_1 + l_1 \cos(\theta_1 + \theta_4) \tag{2.51}$$

$$\frac{d\theta_4}{d\theta_1} = \frac{-s_1 \cos\theta_1 + l_1 \cos(\theta_1 + \theta_4)}{(s_1 \cos\theta_4 - l_1 \cos(\theta_1 + \theta_4))} \tag{2.52}$$

or

$$\frac{d\theta_2}{d\theta_1} = \frac{-s_1 \cos\theta_1 + l_1 \cos(\theta_1 + \theta_2)}{(s_1 \cos\theta_2 - l_1 \cos(\theta_1 + \theta_2))} \tag{2.53}$$

as $\theta_2 = \theta_4$.

The transmission ratio is given by (2.36) and is the rate of change of the input angle, θ_1, with respect to the rate of change of the output angle of the link AC, $180 - \theta_2$.

$$\frac{d(180 - \theta_2)}{d\theta_1} = -\frac{d\theta_2}{d\theta_1} \tag{2.54}$$

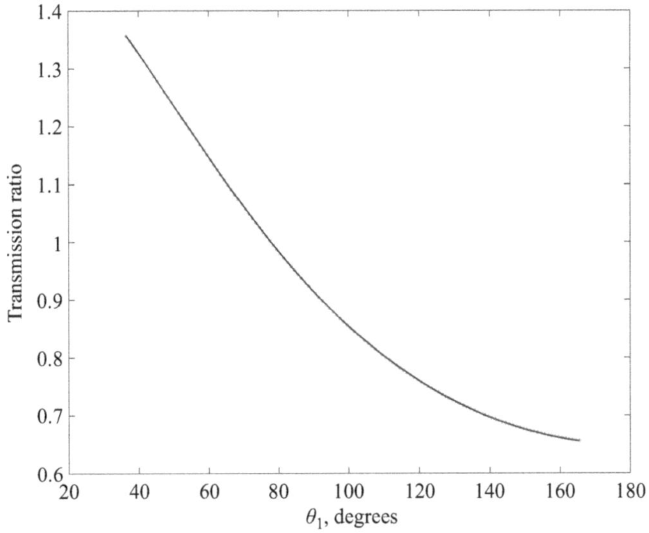

Figure 2.20 Transmission ratio as a function of the input angle, θ_1. The lengths of the links are $l_1 = l_2 = 70.71$ mm and $s_1 = s_2 = 15$ mm

The transmission ratio (plotted in Figure 2.20) is

$$t_r = -\frac{d\theta_2}{d\theta_1} = \frac{s_1 \cos\theta_1 - l_1 \cos(\theta_1 + \theta_2)}{(s_1 \cos\theta_2 - l_1 \cos(\theta_1 + \theta_2))} \tag{2.55}$$

The lengths of the links can be chosen to produce the maximum force for a given input torque. The transmission ratio is unity when the link BC is parallel to the link OA and $\theta_1 = \theta_2 = \theta_3 = \theta_4$.

The fingertip force, F_t, is given by

$$F_t = \frac{T_p}{l_3 t_r} \tag{2.56}$$

where the input torque at the joint O is T_p, t_r is the transmission ratio and l_3 is the length of the fingertip link.

Figure 2.21 shows the normal force output at the tip for a torque input of 1 N·m.

The rotation of the link BC is given by

$$\frac{d\theta_{BC}}{d\theta_1} = \frac{d(180 - \theta_4 + \theta_1)}{d\theta_1} = -\frac{d\theta_4}{d\theta_1} + 1 \tag{2.57}$$

Substituting (2.52) into (2.57)

$$\frac{d\theta_{BC}}{d\theta_1} = \frac{s_1 \cos\theta_1 - l_1 \cos(\theta_1 + \theta_4) + s_1 \cos\theta_4 - l_1 \cos(\theta_1 + \theta_4)}{(s_1 \cos\theta_4 - l_1 \cos(\theta_1 + \theta_4))} \tag{2.58}$$

$$\frac{d\theta_{BC}}{d\theta_1} = \frac{-2l_1 \cos(\theta_1 + \theta_4) + s_1(\cos\theta_1 + \cos\theta_4)}{(s_1 \cos\theta_4 - l_1 \cos(\theta_1 + \theta_4))} \tag{2.59}$$

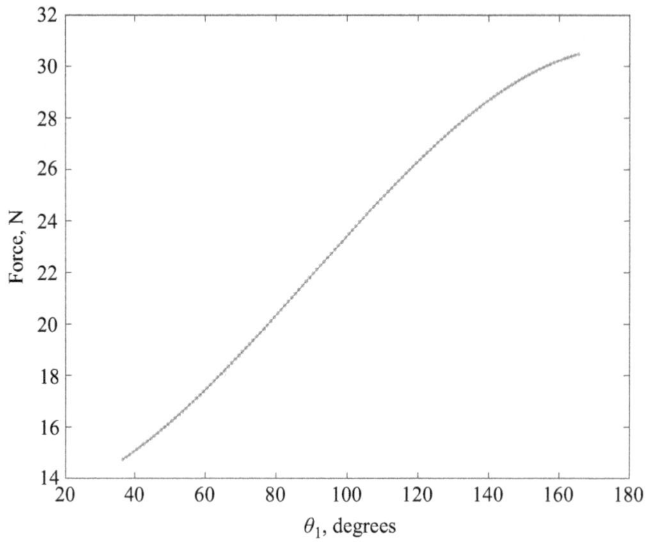

Figure 2.21 Generated force at the fingertip from a constant torque of 1 N·m applied to the link OB in a counterclockwise sense as a function of the input angle, θ_1. The lengths of the links are $l_1 = l_2 = 70.71$ mm and $s_1 = s_2 = 15$ mm

For unequal lengths of the links, the transmission ratio can be determined using the geometric properties of the triangles. In Figure 2.18, the triangles OAC and OBC have the common base, r_1.

Applying the cosine law to these triangles

$$r_1^2 = l_2^2 + s_1^2 - 2l_2s_1\cos\theta_2 \tag{2.60}$$

$$r_1^2 = l_1^2 + s_2^2 - 2l_1s_2\cos\theta_4 \tag{2.61}$$

Similarly, the triangles OAB and ABC have the common base, r_2.

$$r_2^2 = l_1^2 + s_1^2 - 2l_1s_1\cos\theta_1 \tag{2.62}$$

$$r_2^2 = l_2^2 + s_2^2 - 2l_2s_2\cos\theta_3 \tag{2.63}$$

Eliminating ${r_1}^2$ from (2.60) and (2.61) and ${r_2}^2$ from (2.58) and (2.59)

$$l_2^2 + s_1^2 - 2l_2s_1\cos\theta_2 = l_1^2 + s_2^2 - 2l_1s_2\cos\theta_4 \tag{2.64}$$

$$l_1^2 + s_1^2 - 2l_1s_1\cos\theta_1 = l_2^2 + s_2^2 - 2l_2s_2\cos\theta_3 \tag{2.65}$$

Differentiating (2.64) and (2.65) with respect to θ_1

$$-2l_2s_1(-\sin\theta_2)\frac{d\theta_2}{d\theta_1} = -2l_1s_2(-\sin\theta_4)\frac{d\theta_4}{d\theta_1} \tag{2.66}$$

$$-2l_1s_1(-\sin\theta_1) = -2l_2s_2(-\sin\theta_3)\frac{d\theta_3}{d\theta_1} \tag{2.67}$$

Rearranging (2.66) and (2.67)

$$\frac{d\theta_2}{d\theta_1} = \frac{l_1 s_2 \sin\theta_4}{l_2 s_1 \sin\theta_2}\frac{d\theta_4}{d\theta_1} \tag{2.68}$$

$$\frac{d\theta_3}{d\theta_1} = \frac{l_1 s_1 \sin\theta_1}{l_2 s_2 \sin\theta_3} \tag{2.69}$$

$$\frac{d\theta_4}{d\theta_1} = \frac{l_2 s_1 \sin\theta_2}{l_1 s_2 \sin\theta_4}\frac{d\theta_2}{d\theta_1} \tag{2.70}$$

The four angles, θ_1, θ_2, θ_3 and θ_4 are related by

$$\theta_1 + \theta_2 + \theta_{10} = 180 = \theta_3 + \theta_4 + \theta_{10} \tag{2.71}$$

$$\theta_1 + \theta_2 = \theta_3 + \theta_4 \tag{2.72}$$

Differentiating (2.72) with respect to θ_1

$$\frac{d\theta_2}{d\theta_1} = \frac{d\theta_3}{d\theta_1} + \frac{d\theta_4}{d\theta_1} - 1 \tag{2.73}$$

Substituting (2.69) and (2.70) into (2.73)

$$\frac{d\theta_2}{d\theta_1} = \frac{l_1 s_1 \sin\theta_1}{l_2 s_2 \sin\theta_3} + \frac{l_2 s_1 \sin\theta_2}{l_1 s_2 \sin\theta_4}\frac{d\theta_2}{d\theta_1} - 1 \tag{2.74}$$

Rearranging (2.74)

$$\frac{d\theta_2}{d\theta_1} = \frac{\left[\dfrac{l_1 s_1 \sin\theta_1}{l_2 s_2 \sin\theta_3} - 1\right]}{\left[-\dfrac{l_2 s_1 \sin\theta_2}{l_1 s_2 \sin\theta_4} + 1\right]} \tag{2.75}$$

$$\frac{d\theta_2}{d\theta_1} = \frac{\left[\dfrac{l_1 s_1 \sin\theta_1 - l_2 s_2 \sin\theta_3}{l_2 s_2 \sin\theta_3}\right]}{\left[\dfrac{-l_2 s_1 \sin\theta_2 + l_1 s_2 \sin\theta_4}{l_1 s_2 \sin\theta_4}\right]} \tag{2.76}$$

$$\frac{d\theta_2}{d\theta_1} = \frac{l_1 \sin\theta_4 (l_1 s_1 \sin\theta_1 - l_2 s_2 \sin\theta_3)}{l_2 \sin\theta_3 (-l_2 s_1 \sin\theta_2 + l_1 s_2 \sin\theta_4)} \tag{2.77}$$

$$t_r = \frac{d(180 - \theta_2)}{d\theta_1} = -\frac{d\theta_2}{d\theta_1} \tag{2.78}$$

$$t_r = \frac{l_1 \sin\theta_4 (l_1 s_1 \sin\theta_1 - l_2 s_2 \sin\theta_3)}{l_2 \sin\theta_3 (l_2 s_1 \sin\theta_2 - l_1 s_2 \sin\theta_4)} \tag{2.79}$$

With unequal lengths of the links, the transmission ratio is plotted in Figure 2.22. Figure 2.23 shows the normal force output at the tip for a torque input of 1 N·m. Equation (2.79) is not valid for equal lengths where the previous equation should be used (2.55).

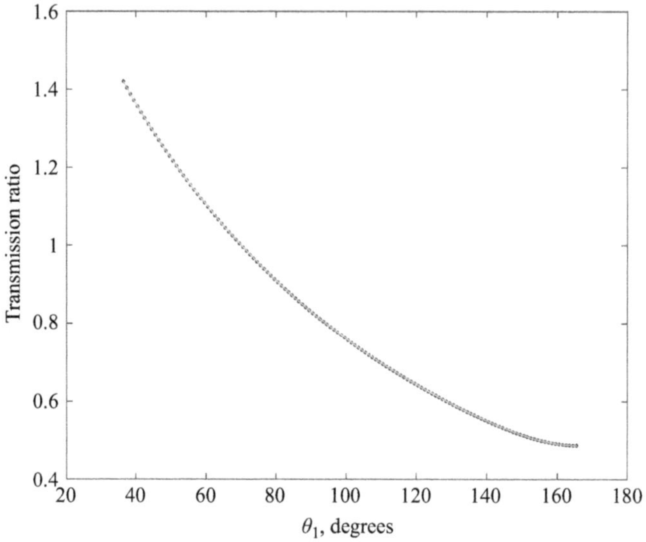

Figure 2.22 Transmission ratio as a function of the input angle, θ_1. The lengths of the links are $l_1 = 68$ mm, $l_2 = 69$ mm, $s_1 = 14$ mm and $s_2 = 16$ mm

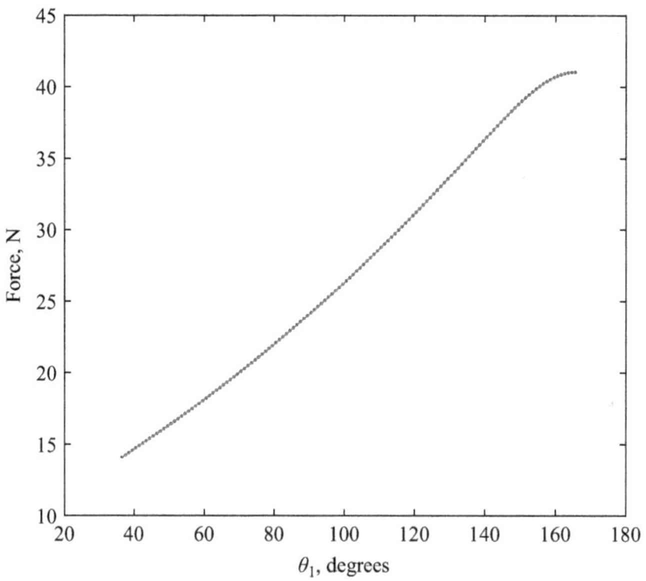

Figure 2.23 Generated force at the fingertip from a constant torque of 1 N·m applied to the link OB in a counterclockwise sense as a function of the input angle, θ_1. The lengths of the links are $l_1 = 68$ mm, $l_2 = 69$ mm, $s_1 = 14$ mm and $s_2 = 16$ mm

For the link BC, differentiating (2.72) with respect to θ_1

$$\frac{d\theta_4}{d\theta_1} = 1 + \frac{d\theta_2}{d\theta_1} - \frac{d\theta_3}{d\theta_1} \tag{2.80}$$

Substituting (2.68) and (2.69) into (2.80)

$$\frac{d\theta_4}{d\theta_1} = 1 + \frac{l_1 s_2 \sin\theta_4}{l_2 s_1 \sin\theta_2}\frac{d\theta_4}{d\theta_1} - \frac{l_1 s_1 \sin\theta_1}{l_2 s_2 \sin\theta_3} \tag{2.81}$$

Rearranging (2.81)

$$\frac{d\theta_4}{d\theta_1} = \frac{\left[\dfrac{l_1 s_1 \sin\theta_1}{l_2 s_2 \sin\theta_3} - 1\right]}{\left[\dfrac{l_1 s_2 \sin\theta_4}{l_2 s_1 \sin\theta_2} - 1\right]} \tag{2.82}$$

$$\frac{d\theta_4}{d\theta_1} = \frac{\left[\dfrac{l_1 s_1 \sin\theta_1 - l_2 s_2 \sin\theta_3}{l_2 s_2 \sin\theta_3}\right]}{\left[\dfrac{l_1 s_2 \sin\theta_4 - l_2 s_1 \sin\theta_2}{l_2 s_1 \sin\theta_2}\right]} \tag{2.83}$$

$$\frac{d\theta_4}{d\theta_1} = \frac{s_1 \sin\theta_2 (l_1 s_1 \sin\theta_1 - l_2 s_2 \sin\theta_3)}{s_2 \sin\theta_3 (l_1 s_2 \sin\theta_4 - l_2 s_1 \sin\theta_2)} \tag{2.84}$$

2.6 Curling fingers and two four-bar linkages

Guo, Lee and Gruver [3, 4] first studied a mechanism with two four-bar linkages for use in artificial hands. Light also used this mechanism [5]. This six-bar linkage is driven by the link OB in Figure 2.24. The four-bar link mechanism shown in

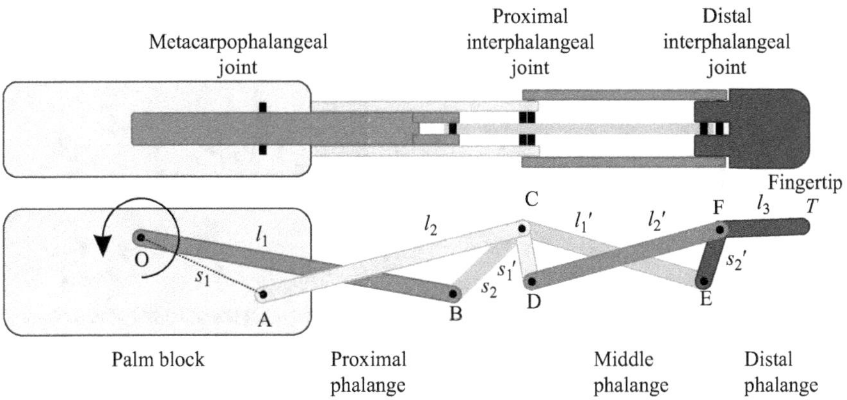

Figure 2.24 Diagrammatic view of a multilink finger with two four-bar linkages. Top and side views

Figure 2.18 can be added to a second set, forming a curling finger that represents all the natural joints and phalanges. This arrangement is shown in Figure 2.24. The links OABC are the first four-bar linkage with CDEF forming the second set. The link EF extends beyond pivot F to the fingertip, *T*. Force is transmitted from the first set to the second set using links ACD and BCE. These links ACD and BCD are solid components that pivot around joint C. Similarly force is transmitted to the fingertip, *T*, via the solid link EFT that pivots around F. An electric drive connected to a shaft at the pivot, O, rotates the link OB in a counterclockwise direction to curl the finger into the palm. Alternatively, link AC can be powered and rotated counterclockwise around pivot A.

In Figure 2.25, the link OB is rotated every 20 degrees and demonstrates the action of the two sets of four-bar linkages. Different curling trajectories of the tip shown in Figure 2.26 can be formed by adjusting the dimensions, l_1, l_2, s_1, s_2, l_1', l_2', s_1', s_2' and l_3 shown in Figure 2.27.

The relationship between the angle of OB with respect to the palm surface (horizontal, *x*-axis) and the tip, *T*, can be determined from two sets of equations of the two mechanisms for OABC and CDEF with the addition of the equations for *T*. A detailed diagram of the joint at C in Figure 2.27 is shown in Figure 2.28 where the constant angle of link ACD is the angle θ_{16} and the constant angle of link BCE is the angle θ_{15}. As the input link, OB, is rotated counterclockwise the angle θ_3 decreases. As ACD and BCE are solid components, then θ_{15} and θ_{16} are constant. The rotation of OB causes the input angle, θ_3', to the second four-bar mechanism to also decrease, resulting a curling action of the finger.

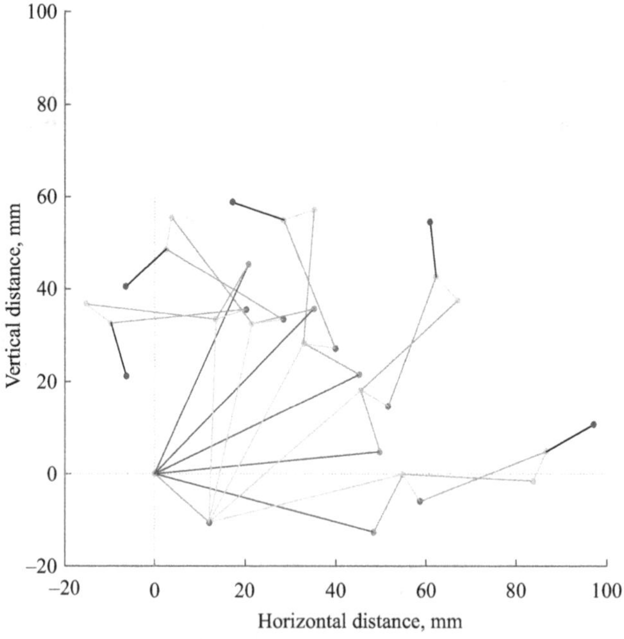

Figure 2.25 Multiple joint links showing trajectories every 20 degrees from 0 to 80-degree rotation of link OB

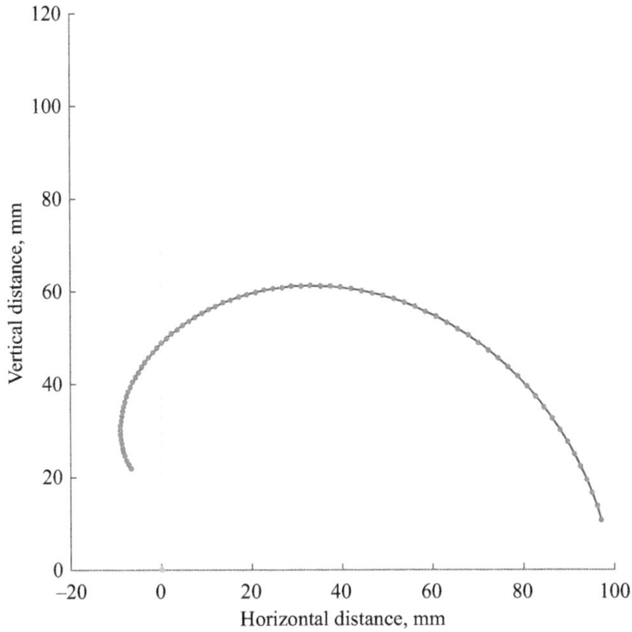

Figure 2.26 Multiple joint links showing trajectory of the tip every 1 degree from 0 to 80-degree rotation of link OB

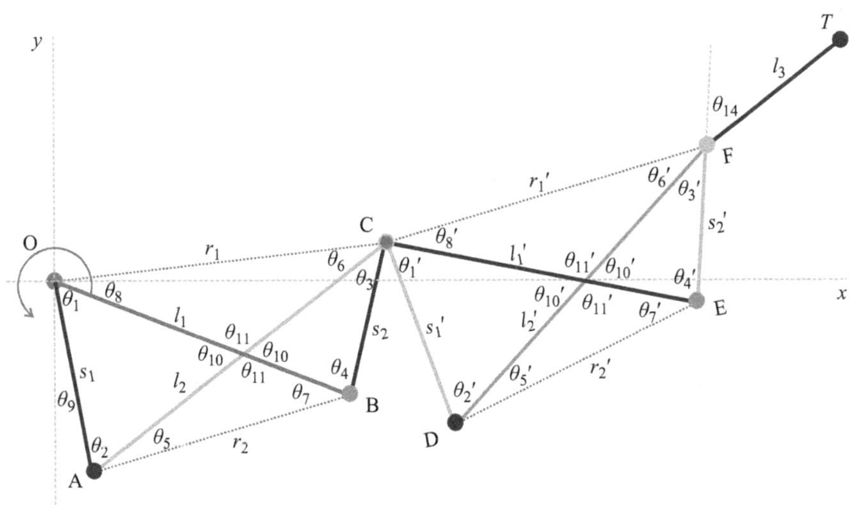

Figure 2.27 Diagram of a two coupled sets a four-bar linkage with crossed links showing dimensions and angles

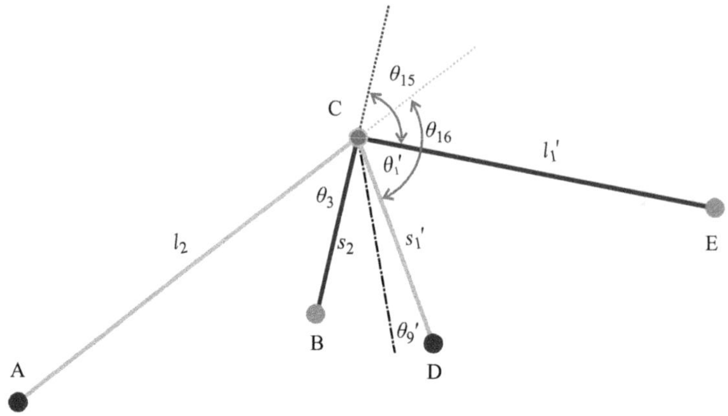

Figure 2.28 Detail of joint C showing the angles between links ACD and BCE

The relationship between the angle, θ_3, of the first set of links and the angle, θ_1' of the second set is given by

$$\theta_1' = \theta_3 + \theta_{16} - \theta_{15} \tag{2.85}$$

The orientation of link AC in the *x-y* plane, which is connected to CD, is

$$\theta_{AC} = \tan^{-1}\frac{y_C - y_B}{x_C - x_B} \tag{2.86}$$

Then the angle of the second set of links is

$$\theta_9' = \theta_{AC} - \theta_{16} \tag{2.87}$$

2.7 Thumb

The natural thumb has five degrees of freedom. For an artificial thumb a simple powered stick is all that is required to flex and extend into the palm since once in position the fingers can be moved to form a grip. An improvement is to power the rotation of the thumb about the metacarpal axis.

2.8 Actuators

Small DC motors with gearboxes can be used to power fingers and thumbs. The rotation of the shaft of a gearbox can be translated to linear motion in several ways. A small motor with a gearbox made from planetary gears can rotate the link OB in Figures 2.18 and 2.27. However, even if the gearbox ratio is high by applying force to the fingertip the motor can be backdriven resulting in loss of grip if the motor is not powered. However, using a worm-wheel drive eliminates the need for a locking mechanism when power is removed from the motor (Figure 2.29).

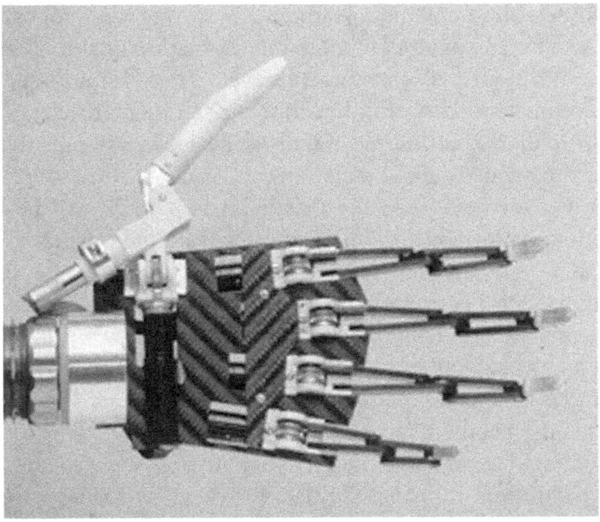

Figure 2.29 *A handmade from carbon fibre showing the worm-wheel drives at the metacarpophalangeal joints. The motor and gearboxes are on the located on the dorsal surface of the palm plate. The thumb is actuated by another worm-wheel drive*

A lead screw mechanism also translates the rotary motion into linear motion and can lock a finger in position when the motor is disconnected [6].

The electrical energy from a battery can be converted to mechanical energy using a small DC motor to power a finger or thumb. The rotational velocity of the motor is high, and a gearbox is needed to reduce the velocity to about 0.25 revolutions per second or less. This velocity corresponds to a rotation of the proximal phalange by 90 degrees in one second. Two stages of reduction in the velocity are required.

$$w_{pp} = \frac{w_m}{R_b R_{ww}} \tag{2.88}$$

where w_{pp} is the angular velocity of the proximal joint, R_b is the motor gearbox ratio, R_{ww} is the worm-wheel ratio and w_m is the motor angular velocity.

The corresponding torque equation is

$$T_{pp} = R_b R_{ww} T_m \tag{2.89}$$

where T_{pp} is the torque at the proximal joint and T_m the developed motor torque.

A finger should close into the palm of a hand in less than one second. A longer time is not acceptable to the user of an artificial hand, and this parameter sets a boundary condition for the design of the actuator in the selection of a suitable motor and gearbox ratios. In practice, there are inefficiencies in the mechanisms that increase the closing time from the ideal design and reduce the fingertip force.

From experiments with designs of finger mechanisms at full rated voltage, small DC motors tend to rotate close to their no-load angular velocity. This parameter then sets the combined gearbox and worm-wheel ratios, i.e., $R_b R_{ww}$, which in turn sets the maximum output torque at the proximal joint and maximum fingertip force. When stalled, a motor can develop maximum torque. This torque can be used to estimate the fingertip force for a given finger mechanism. However, the temperature will rise inside the motor as the power dissipation is armature resistance times the square of the stall current. A motor will not be able to withstand the heating indefinitely, so the maximum grip force will be time limited. Another possibility is to model the heat transfer from the interior of the motor to ambient air and to estimate the core temperature of the motor. A first-order differential equation with decaying exponential time functions is a suitable model. The time constants are calculated using the manufacturer's thermal parameters for the motor and an estimate of ambient temperature. The maximum duration for the peak force can be calculated, and the current interrupted before the motor temperature exceeds its specified value.

The selection of a suitable motor, to power a mechanism, requires the inspection of parameters from lists of data provided by manufactures. Of prime importance is that a motor should have a low mass, but this may result in the selection of one that has either a low rotational velocity or a low torque. A motor should have high-stall torque for gripping and a high no-load speed for fast movement of fingers and thumbs. These desired specifications conflict. Heavy motors are more powerful, generating high torque but with lower velocities. Alternatively, a low mass motor may have a high rotational velocity but low torque.

The parameters of mass, stall torque and no-load rotational velocity are shown in the scatter plots of Figures 2.30 and 2.31. At the upper left part of the plots are

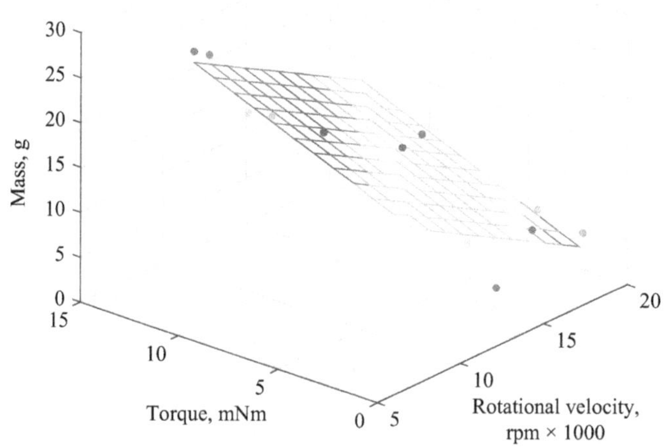

Figure 2.30 The three important variables of mass, stall torque and no-load rotational velocity

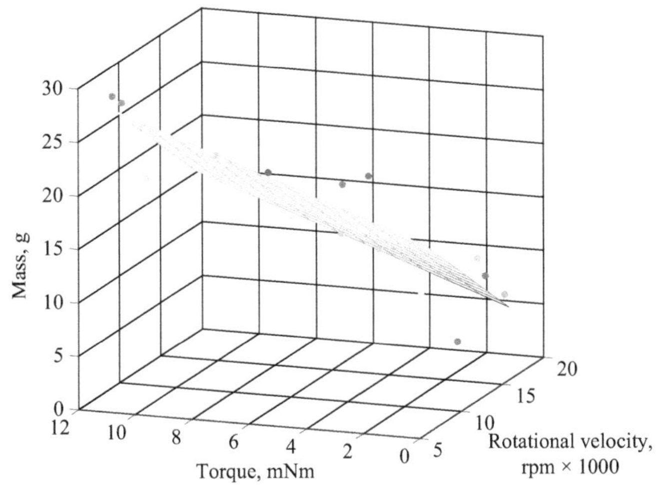

Figure 2.31 A different view of the three important variables of mass, stall torque and no-load rotational velocity

motors with high masses and torque but with low velocities. On the other end of the range in the lower right of the plot are motors with high velocities and low mass but low torque. In general, it is better to choose a motor that has a low mass where there is then a compromise between velocity and torque. A slow closing velocity of a finger will not be tolerated, so the parameter that may be restricted is grip force.

From the left to right in Figure 2.32, as the mass increases the velocity decreases and the torque increases. In Figure 2.33, the torque increases as the mass increases. In Figure 2.34, the velocity decreases as the mass increases. The regression lines on the plots show the general trends; individual motors may a have better performance, e.g., the two motors towards the centre of Figure 2.32 have a higher velocity for a torque of approximately 5 mNm.

For a worm-wheel drive, a desirable ratio is about 20:1, so that on removal of power a finger cannot be backdriven and an object will be held in the hand. The gearbox connecting the motor to the worm-wheel also may have restrictions such as the maximum rotational speed and torque.

The selection of a motor, gearbox and worm wheel is a multi-parameter problem.

Childress proposed a mechanism that has a high velocity and low force when the fingers are needed to flex or extend quickly and a high force at low velocities when contact is made with an object and gripping is needed [7]. This desirable characteristic is achieved with two motors and gearboxes driving the finger mechanism. A high gear ratio is used for rapid movement and a low ratio for force generation. The disadvantage of this method is the added complexity and mass from two mechanisms.

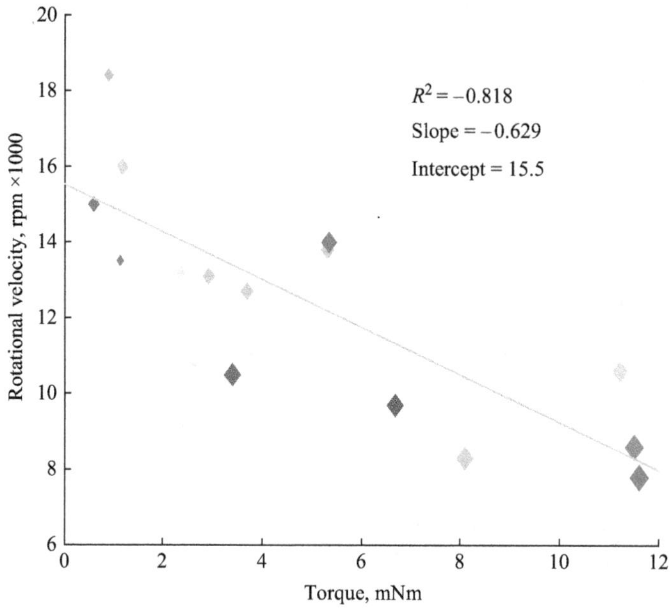

Figure 2.32 No-load rotational velocity against stall torque. The area of each data point is in proportion to the mass of the motor

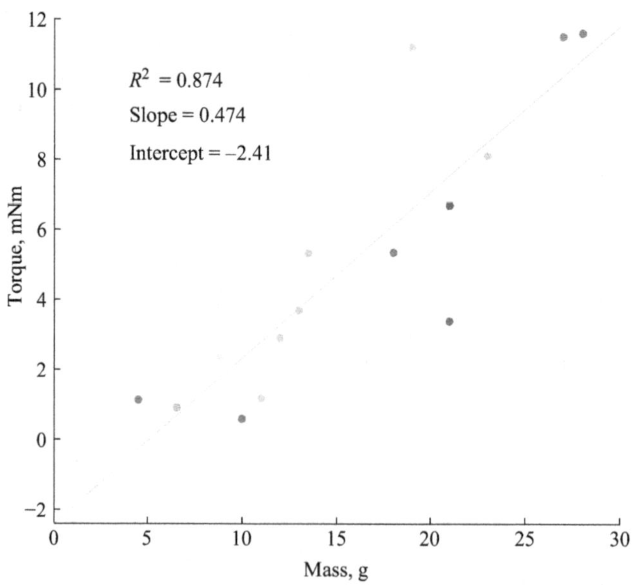

Figure 2.33 Stall torque against mass

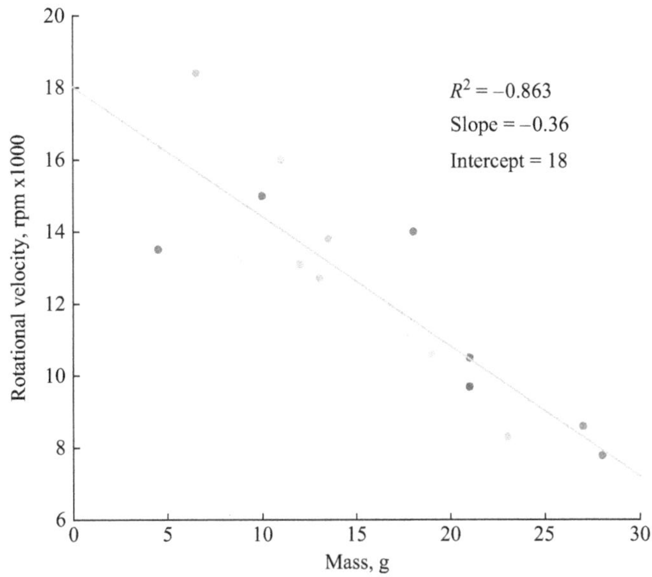

Figure 2.34 No-load rotational velocity against mass

2.9 Summary

A wide variety of mechanisms are available for the mechanical design of fingers and thumbs. A simple driven link with one actuator offers a lightweight and robust design with limited grip postures. The addition of multiple links in a four-bar linkage results in a more natural curling finger action. Adding a second four-bar linkage allows for rotation about each of the joints but with added complexity. Force generation is a nonlinear function of the input joint angle, and the finger links can be chosen for a desired force profile. Some actuators lock when there is no power input ensuring a stable object grip and power saving, otherwise, an electromechanical brake is needed. The mechanical parts can be made with lightweight metal alloys for robustness but where possible should be made from low-density polymers. There is a balance to make between a design that rapidly moves the fingers, with a high gear ratio, and one where a high grip force is achieved with a low gear ratio.

References

1 Moore D. *Development of a Multifunctional Adaptive Hand Prosthesis*, PhD thesis, University of Southampton, 1981

2 Rothenhofer G., Walsh C., and Slocum A. 'Transmission ratio based analysis and robust design of mechanisms', *Precision Engineering*, 2010;**34**:790–797

3 Guo, G., Lee, T. T., and Gruver W. A. 'Design of a planar multijointed prosthetic finger mechanism', *Transactions of the ASME in Design Engineering*, 1990;**26**:165–170
4 Guo G. and Gruver W. A. 'Optimal design of a six bar linkage with 1 DOF for an anthropomorphic three-jointed finger mechanism', *Proceedings of the Institution of Mechanical Engineers*, 1993;**207**:185–190
5 Light C. M. *An Intelligent Hand Prosthesis and Evaluation of Pathological and Prosthetic Hand Function*, PhD thesis, University of Southampton, 2000
6 Kyberd P. J. *Algorithmic Control of a Multifunction Hand Prosthesis*, PhD thesis, University of Southampton, 1990
7 Childress D. S. 'An approach to powered grasp', *Proceedings of the Fourth International Symposium on External Control of Human Extremities*, Dubrovnik, Yugoslavia, 1973, 159–167

Chapter 3
Sensors

3.1 Characteristics

There are many sensors that measure physical variables such as temperature with different technologies in a wide range of applications. The sensors used in the automotive and aerospace industries have demanding requirements in hostile environments. These sensors can find their way into artificial hands, e.g., the accelerometers used for crash detection in vehicles. However, some of these sensors are too large to fit into a hand or consume too much electrical power and are not suitable. Sensors for artificial hands have a demanding specification as shown in Figure 3.1.

Sensors are essential components in any design of artificial hands to give warning signals to the wearer of a prosthesis or inform an electronic controller. When an object is too hot or too cold, it can be quickly released from the hand to avoid damage to the person or glove. Also the operation of a hand is made easier when a sensor provides information to form a closed-loop control system. Sensing of force, finger position, object slip, surface texture and temperature can best be achieved with the low-cost technology of screen printing. Traditional metal materials have been used to construct the mechanical parts of a hand, but there is a newer requirement to develop sensors that can be easily mounted on new polymer materials.

There are three basic electrical properties of an electronic circuit that can be varied to make a sensor. A resistor dissipates energy compared to a capacitance where energy can be stored in an electric field and an inductor where energy is stored in a magnetic field. The properties of these components are given below.

A resistor (resistance, R) is governed by Ohm's Law.

$$v = Ri \tag{3.1}$$

Capacitor (capacitance, C)

$$v = \frac{1}{C}\int i\,dt \quad i = C\frac{dv}{dt} \quad \Delta I = C\frac{\Delta V}{\Delta t} \tag{3.2}$$

Inductor (inductance, L)

$$i = \frac{1}{L}\int v\,dt \quad v = L\frac{di}{dt} \quad \Delta V = L\frac{\Delta I}{\Delta t} \tag{3.3}$$

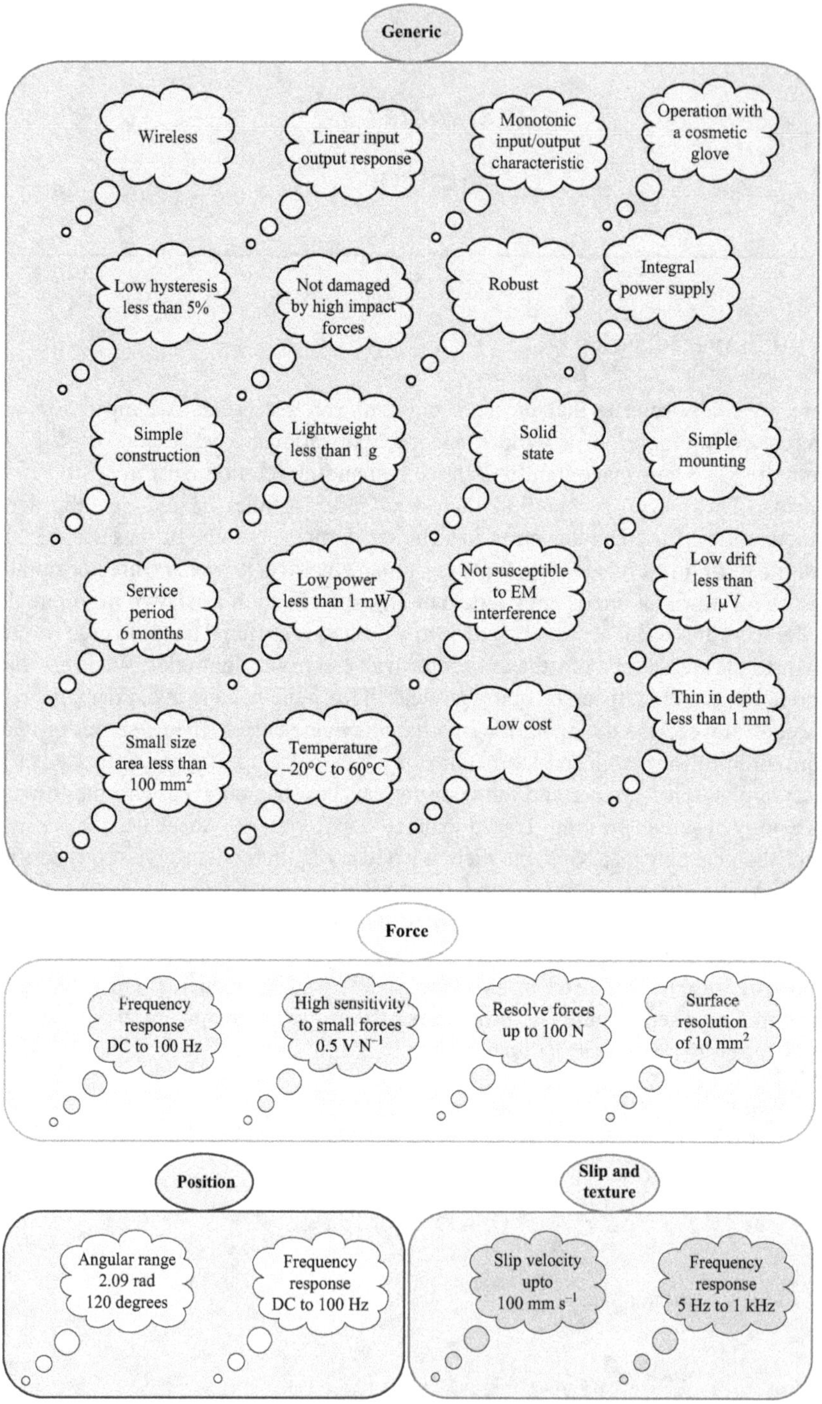

Figure 3.1 Generic characteristics for sensors used in artificial hands

There are various standard techniques to measure the resistance, capacitance or inductance of a sensor. If the variable to be measured such as force, m, affects one of these three parameters, then

$$m = f(R) \quad or \quad m = f(C) \quad or \quad m = f(L) \tag{3.4}$$

where f is a linear or monotonic function. Some possible functions for resistance, R, are shown in Table 3.1.

Table 3.1 Functions for m

Linear	$m = A_1 + A_2 R$	(3.5)
Quadratic	$m = A_1 + A_2 R + A_3 R^2$	(3.6)
Inverse	$m = A_1 \left(\frac{1}{(R - A_2)} - A_3 \right)$	(3.7)
Exponential	$m = A_1 + A_2 \exp(\pm A_3 R)$	(3.8)
Logarithmic	$m = A_1 + A_2 \ln(A_3 R)$	(3.9)

A linear characteristic is desirable for most sensor applications, but sometimes a nonlinear characteristic can have advantages such as a high sensitivity at low values. An example of the benefit of high sensitivity occurs in the holding of a delicate object where good control over small forces is required to avoid damaging the object.

3.2 Forces sensors

3.2.1 Strain gauge

Strain gauges are commonly made from metal foils where their resistance varies as they are stretched or compressed. The resistivity of the material, ρ, determines the measured resistance that depends on the length, l, and the cross-sectional area, a.

$$R = \frac{\rho l}{a} \tag{3.10}$$

Changes in length and area result in a change in resistance. Also there may be changes in the resistivity which is a property called piezoresistance. The typical strain gauge is a thin and rectangular sheet that is elongated on the application of a force, f, shown in Figure 3.2. The thickness of the sheet decreases as does the width. Reversing the direction of the force compresses the material and decreases the length, increases the thickness and increases the width. A force can also be applied across the sensor, i.e., in the z direction as shown in Figure 3.3. A sensor used in this configuration can detect the normal force applied to the planar skin surface.

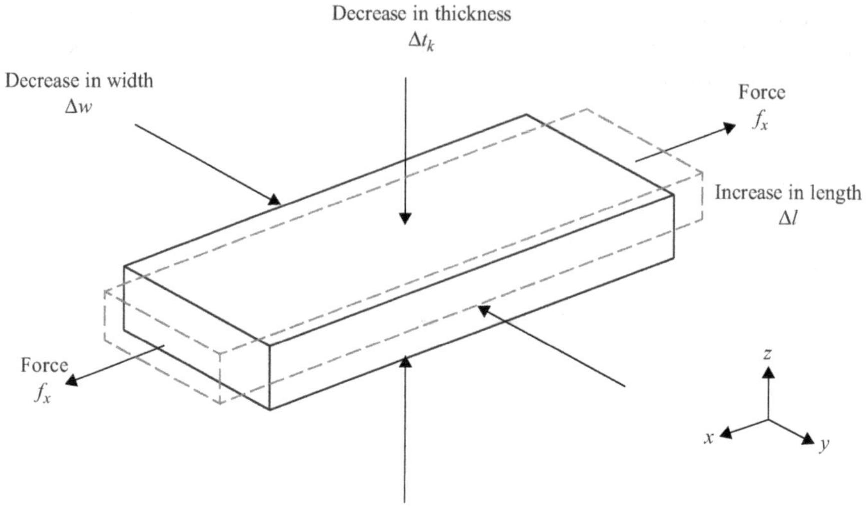

Figure 3.2 A force applied in the x direction causes an increase in the length, a, decrease in thickness (z direction) and a decrease in width (y direction)

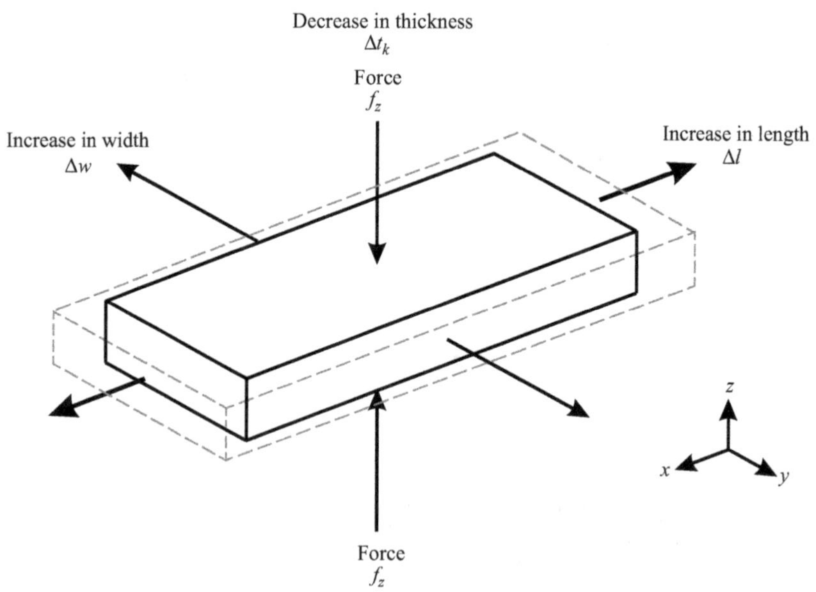

Figure 3.3 A force applied in the z direction causes an increase in the length (x direction), a decrease in thickness (z direction) and an increase in width (y direction)

The strain, ε, for a change in length of Δl, along the x direction in Figure 3.2 is

$$\varepsilon = \frac{\Delta l}{l} \tag{3.11}$$

or

$$l = l + \varepsilon l = l(1 + \varepsilon) \tag{3.12}$$

The resistance is

$$R = \frac{\rho\, l(1 + \varepsilon)}{a} \tag{3.13}$$

$$R(\varepsilon) = \frac{\rho(\varepsilon) l(\varepsilon)}{a(\varepsilon)} = f(\varepsilon) \tag{3.14}$$

$$\frac{dR}{d\varepsilon} = \frac{\partial f}{\partial l}\frac{dl}{d\varepsilon} + \frac{\partial f}{\partial a}\frac{da}{d\varepsilon} + \frac{\partial f}{\partial \rho}\frac{d\rho}{d\varepsilon} \tag{3.15}$$

$$\frac{dR}{d\varepsilon} = \frac{\rho}{a}\frac{dl}{d\varepsilon} - \frac{\rho}{la^2}\frac{da}{d\varepsilon} + \frac{l}{a}\frac{d\rho}{d\varepsilon} \tag{3.16}$$

or

$$\frac{1}{R}\frac{dR}{d\varepsilon} = \frac{1}{l}\frac{dl}{d\varepsilon} - \frac{1}{a}\frac{da}{d\varepsilon} + \frac{1}{\rho}\frac{d\rho}{d\varepsilon} \tag{3.17}$$

A typical metal foil gauge in planar view is illustrated in Figure 3.4.

Strain gauges are typically used with a cantilever beam (Figure 3.5). The metal foil of the strain gauge is mounted on a thin and insulating material that is then glued to the metal beam with an adhesive such as epoxy resin or cyanoacrylate. The attachment requires careful preparation of the metal beam surface to remove any contamination. The beam is made smooth with a fine grade of emery cloth and degreased. The aim is to attach the sensor securely to the beam so as the metal of the beam is strained and a corresponding strain is induced in the metal foil. A thin layer of adhesive allows for the stretching or compressing of the beam to be transmitted to the strain gauge foil. A thick layer causes a loss of sensitivity as it deforms and absorbs the strain, which is then not transmitted to the gauge.

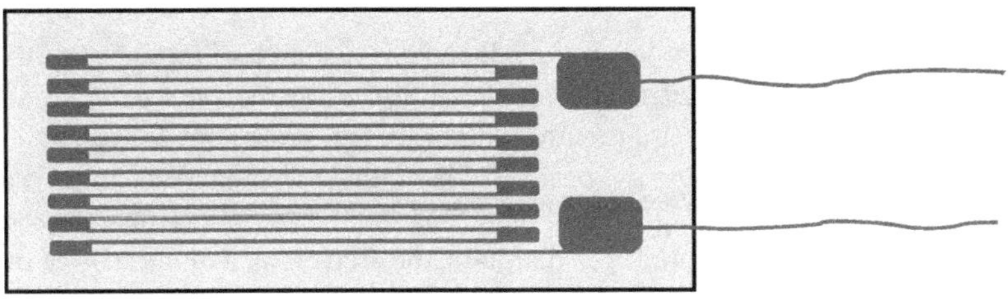

Figure 3.4 Illustration of a typical metal foil strain gauge showing parallel wires on a thin and insulating base with connecting wires

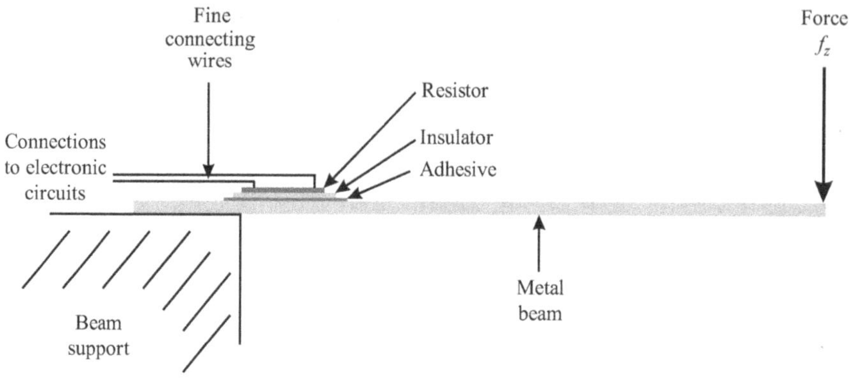

Figure 3.5 Diagrammatic layout of a cantilever beam sensor

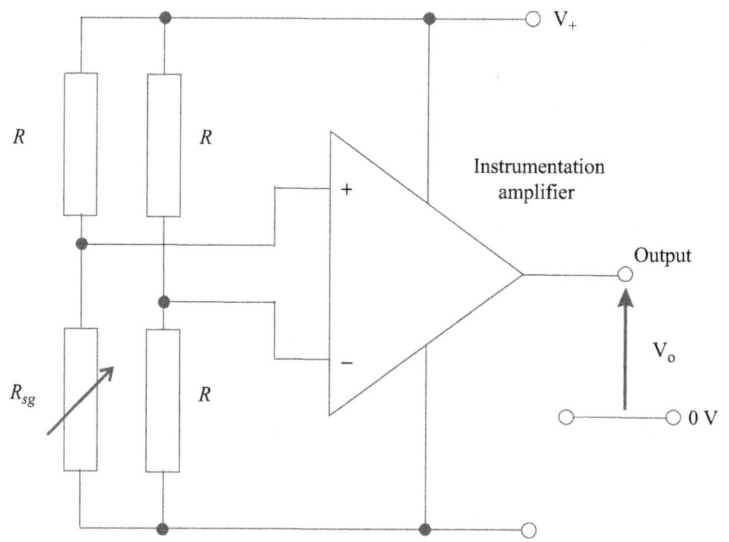

Figure 3.6 Amplifier circuit for a single strain gauge with resistance, R_{sg}

Also, the presence of air bubbles in the adhesive is a source of loss of sensitively. An instrumentation amplifier is used to convert the strain into a voltage signal (Figure 3.6). Three resistors are required that have the same nominal resistance as the unstrained strain gauge. As the beam is flexed, there is an increase in resistance of the strain gauge. The voltage output increases since the two resistors attached to the inverting input of the amplifier maintain the mid-point voltage (0 V) of the power supply (V+ and V−).

Strain gauges are usually used in pairs (top and bottom sensors in Figure 3.7). As the applied force, f_z, deflects the free end of the beam down, the top strain gauge

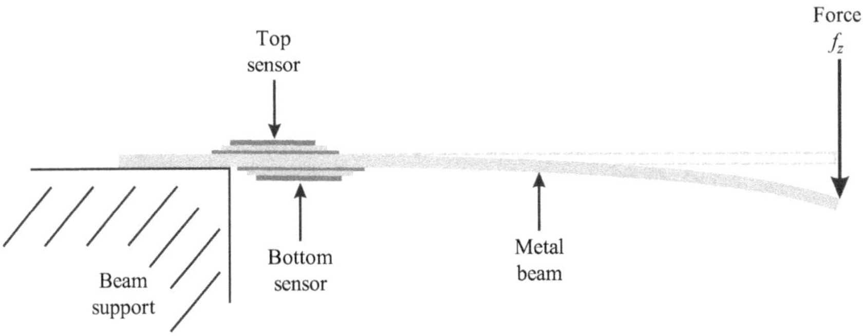

Figure 3.7 Bending of a cantilever beam with two sensors attached to the top and bottom

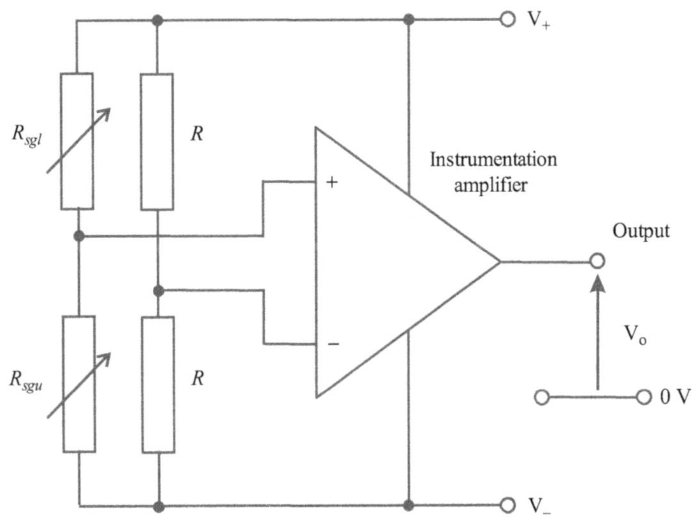

Figure 3.8 Amplifier circuit for two strain gauges with resistances, R_{sgl} and R_{sgu}

is stretched while a second gauge located on the lower surface experiences a compression. This arrangement of sensors has some advantages compared to the single sensor in Figure 3.5. The amplifier circuit for this arrangement of sensors is shown in Figure 3.8. The upper gauge resistance decreases, while the resistance of the lower gauge increases. If the two gauges have similar characteristics, then there is approximately twice the sensitivity compared to the circuit with a single gauge. Also with two gauges, if the ambient temperature changes, then there is some compensation of any drift in the sensor characteristics. If there is an increase in the resistance of one sensor due to a change in ambient temperature, then there will be

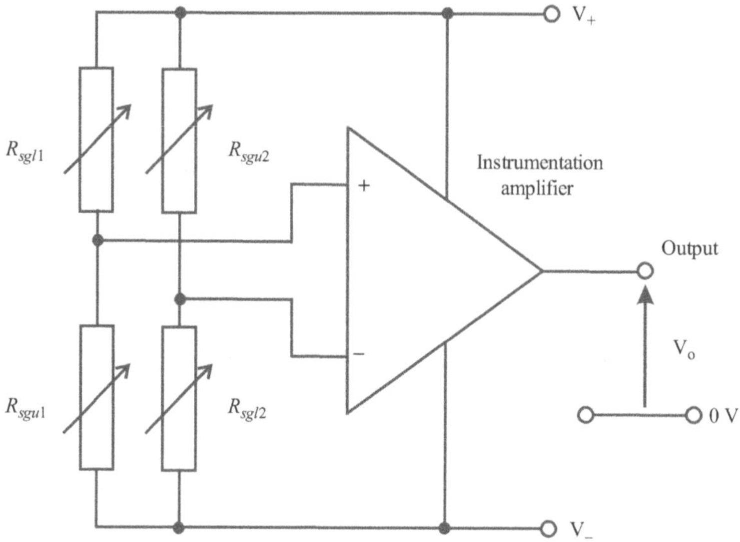

Figure 3.9 Amplifier circuit for four strain gauges with resistances, R_{sgl1}, R_{sgu1}, R_{sgu2} and R_{sgl2}. The two gauges on the top are R_{sgu1} and R_{sgu2} that strained in the opposite sense to the bottom gauges, R_{sgl1} and R_{sgl2}

a corresponding increase in the resistance of the second sensor, which will mitigate the effects of temperature drift from the use of one sensor on its own.

A further refinement of the circuits shown in Figures 3.6 and 3.8 is where four sensors are used in a bridge circuit; two that are stretched and two that are compressed (Figure 3.9). Here the polarity of the sensors is matched to the increases and decreases of the resistance of the gauges to provide maximum sensitivity. For example, the resistances of R_{sgl1} and R_{sgl2} decrease when those of R_{sgu1} and R_{sgu2} increase for a positive application of force.

Metal foil strain gauges have a gauge factor of about two, whereas piezoresistive strain gauges have much higher gauge factors that can be as high as ten. Piezoresistive gauges therefore have a better sensitivity compared to the metal foil types. Figure 3.10 shows an example of the use of piezoresistive materials in a fingertip sensor. These sensors have been made using screen printing where the sensor materials are applied in ink form directly onto the substrate surface, in this case a fingertip. The inks are applied in layers (Figure 3.11). The first layer is an insulating dielectric followed by the resistive layer and then the conductive connections at each end. At each stage a separate mask is used and the assembly heated in an oven at a high temperature. With this technology the adhesive layer shown in Figure 3.5 is not required leading to a more sensitive and robust design. These sensors have the added advantage of being a low-cost solution [1–6]. The principles of amplification are the same as for the metal foil strain gauges (Figures 3.6–3.9).

A strain gauge is attached to the substrate, which for an artificial finger can be made from different materials such as a metal alloy or a plastic. For ceramic

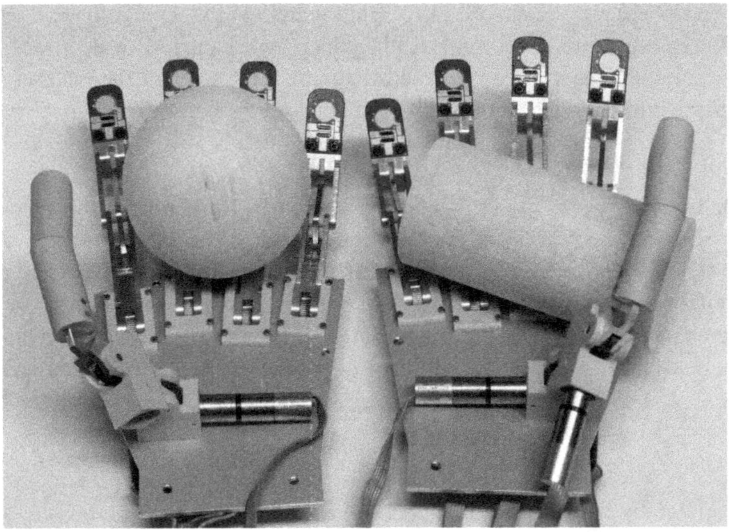

Figure 3.10 Fingertip sensors on a hand [1–4]. The two small black rectangles on each tip are piezoresistive sensors

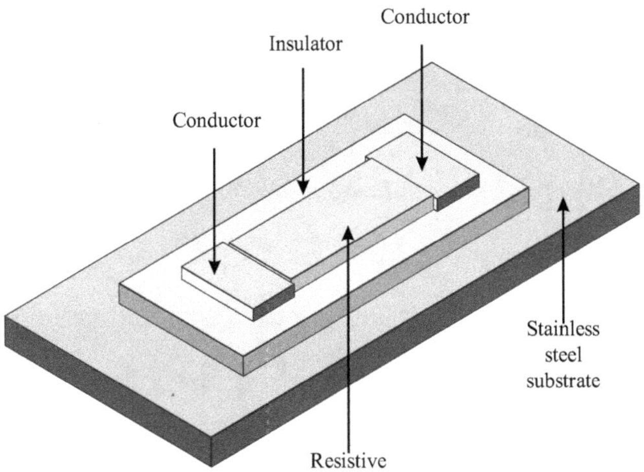

Figure 3.11 Diagrammatic layout of a piezoresistive strain gauge mounted on a steel substrate

piezoresistors a high firing temperature limits the viable material to metals that can withstand these temperatures, such as stainless steels although these come with the disadvantage of a high density [1–6]. Metal foil gauges are designed to be used with aluminium or steel structures. There is an increasing use of polymer materials for the structural components of a hand as they are lightweight, but then there is a need to form sensors that can be made from materials that can withstand less high temperatures (up to about 200°C). Rather than use metal foil or ceramics, piezoresistive polymer materials are needed that can form sensors for integration into fingertips or other hand structures.

3.2.2 Force-sensitive resistors

A conductive polymer is used in the manufacture of a force-sensitive resistor (FSR) whose resistance decreases on the application of a force. These sensors are thin discs or squares and are made in a range of sizes. Attachment with adhesive to the surface of a finger or palm of an artificial hand is straight forward.

The characteristic of an FSR is not linear (Figure 3.12) where the relationship between resistance, r and applied force, f, is governed by the following equation.

$$\frac{1}{(r - R_o)} = S_1 + S_2 f \tag{3.18}$$

or

$$r = R_o + \frac{1}{(S_1 + S_2 f)} \tag{3.19}$$

where, R_o, S_1 and S_2 are parameters.

The derivative of resistance with force is

$$\frac{dr}{df} = -\frac{S_2}{(S_2 + S_2 f)} \tag{3.20}$$

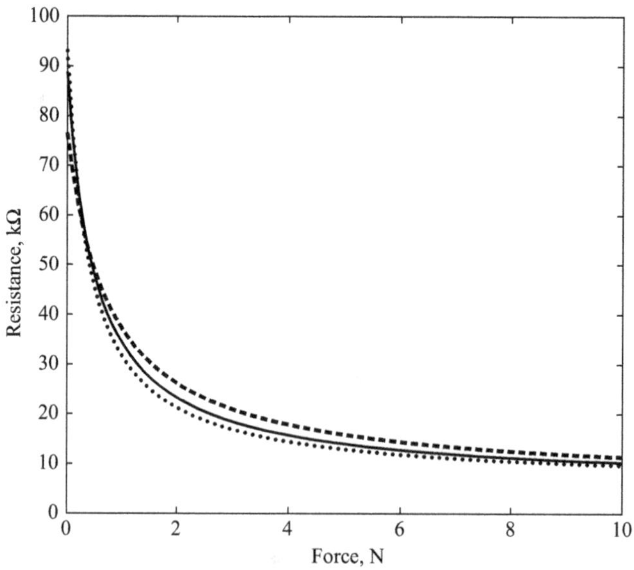

Figure 3.12 Experimental characteristics of an FSR. The top dashed curve is for increasing force and the bottom dotted curve is for decreasing force. The middle continuous curve is the mean of the two characteristics

This nonlinear relationship has the advantage of more sensitivity at low forces (Figure 3.13). However, there is a large hysteresis in the characteristic as shown in Figure 3.12. Increasing the force, from zero, results in higher values of resistance compared to unloading the sensor back to no load. At high forces the sensitivity is low and an estimation of force from a measurement of resistance is not very accurate; above 6 N in Figures 3.12 and 3.13 the characteristic is flat.

The initial resistance at no force is

$$r = R_o + \frac{1}{S_1} \tag{3.21}$$

For the data shown in Figure 3.12, the resistance starts from 93 kΩ on increasing the force and returns to 77 kΩ on reducing the force from 10 N back down to zero.

The amplifier circuit, shown in Figure 3.6, converts the change in resistance, r, into an estimate of the applied force, f. (In Figure 3.6, R_{sg} is the resistance r.)

3.2.3 *Optical*

A force sensor can be made using opto-electronics [7]. The transmitting light source typically operates in the infrared of the light spectrum and is combined with a matched detector. A small light emitting diode (LED) and photodiode can be used to form a sensor (Figure 3.14). An aluminium frame is also needed to house the transmitter and detector with a small plastic tube in the

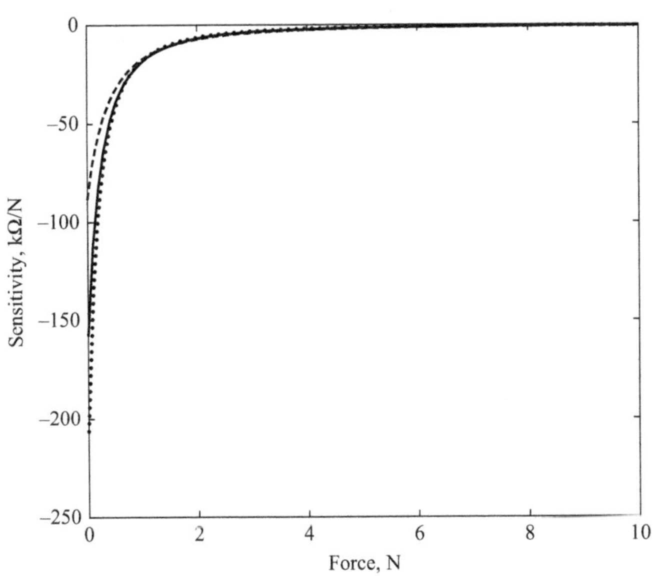

Figure 3.13 Sensitivity characteristics of an FSR. The top dashed curve is for increasing force and the bottom dotted curve is for decreasing force. The middle continuous curve is the mean of the two characteristics

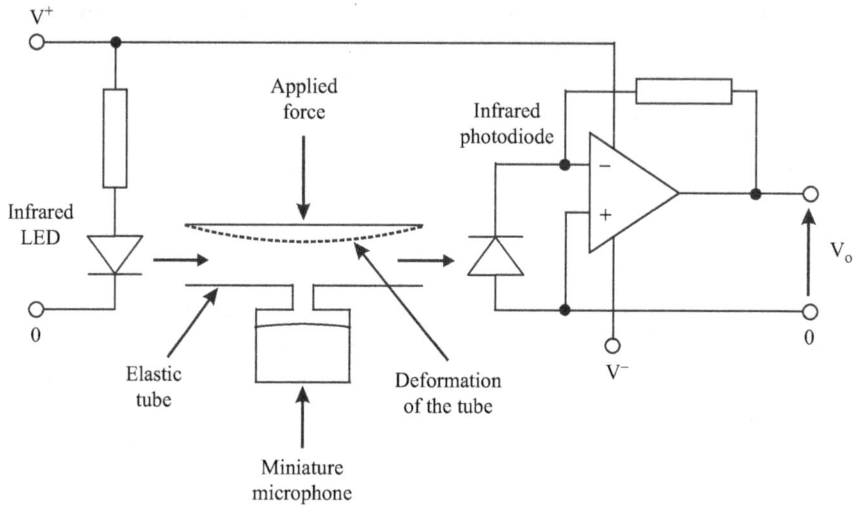

Figure 3.14 Opto-electronic force sensor and slip/texture detection using a microphone

optical path. The cross-sectional area of the tube and light through the tube are reduced when a force is applied via a plunger mounted in the aluminium frame. A change in the transmitted light is detected by the photodiode. The characteristic of this sensor is nonlinear but monotonic. A disadvantage of using opto-electronics is the high power consumption compared to other methods. The average power dissipated in the transmitting LED can be reduced by passing current pulses through the diode instead of a DC current, but this complication requires a clock operating above 1 kHz and a counter to produce the desired pulse width. As shown in Figure 3.14 is a small miniature microphone of the type found in hearing aids, and an amplifier can be connected to the assembly and used to detect slip and texture information.

3.2.4 Capacitance

The variation of capacitance between two conductive surfaces can be put to good effect to form a force sensor. The standard equation for a parallel plate capacitor is given by the following equation.

$$C = \frac{\varepsilon_o \varepsilon_r a}{t_k} \tag{3.22}$$

where ε_o is the permittivity of free space, ε_r is the dielectric constant of the material between the two plates, 'a' the area and t_k is the thickness of the material or distance separating the plates. A force sensor can be made by separating the plates with a material that acts as both a spring and dielectric. As the material is deformed under the application of a force, the capacitance will vary and can be measured.

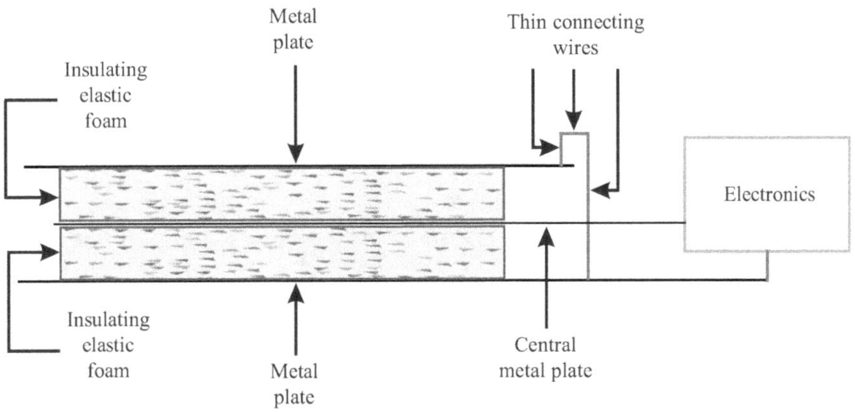

Figure 3.15 Schematic diagram of a capacitive force sensor

For an elastic material with no hysteresis the applied force and distance between the two plates are related by

$$f = k_e(t_{ko} - t_k) \tag{3.23}$$

where k_e is a constant and t_{ko} is the separation when there is no force.

Eliminating t_k from (1.21) and (1.22) gives

$$C = \frac{\varepsilon_o \varepsilon_r a k_e}{(k_e t_{ko} - f)} \tag{3.24}$$

The capacitance is thus an inverse function of the applied force.

A sensor can be made using three plates rather than two as shown in Figure 3.15. This arrangement, where the top and bottom plates are electrically connected, reduces the effects of interference signals.

There are several tried and tested circuits to estimate the capacitance of a component. However for this application, the challenge is that the magnitude of the capacitance is only a few picofarads or less. There are techniques to measure changes in capacitance that are several orders of magnitude less than a picofarad, but they do not estimate the *absolute* value. One practical circuit is shown in Figure 3.16. A square wave output is produced whose frequency decreases with increasing force and has the experimental relationship

$$\omega = A_1 - A_2 f^{A_3} \tag{3.25}$$

where A_1, A_2 and A_3 are parameters.

The sensitivity is better at low forces where the slope of (3.25) is

$$\frac{d\omega}{df} = -A_2 A_3 f^{(A_3 - 1)} \tag{3.26}$$

The parameter A_3 is less than one so the slope decreases with increasing force.

The elastic material separating the plates should have good elastic properties, i.e., no hysteresis. Also it should have a high dielectric constant so as to have a

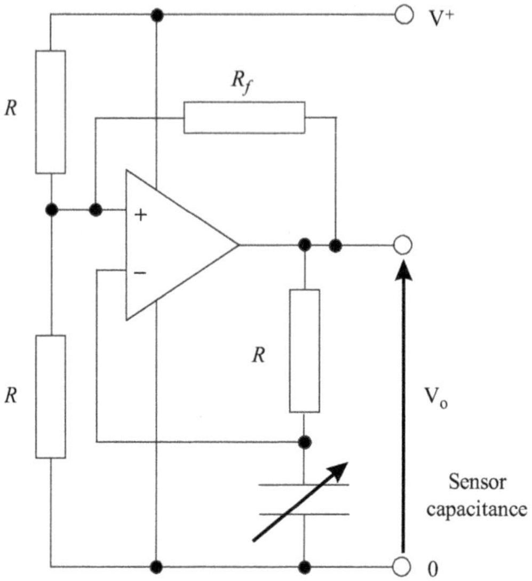

Figure 3.16 Oscillator circuit for detecting the capacitance of a force sensor

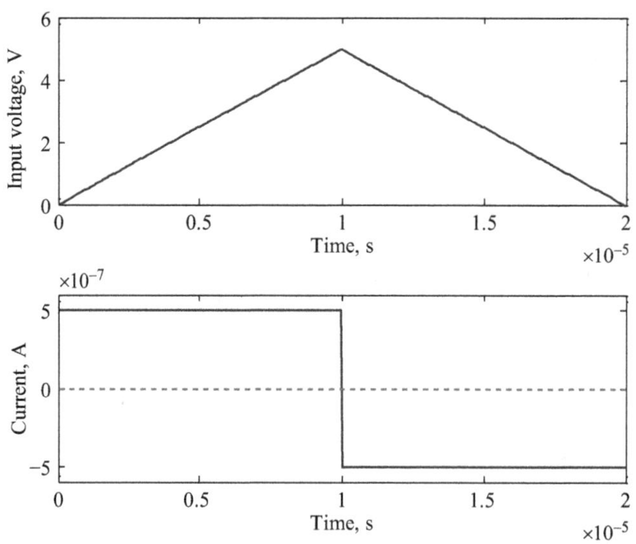

Figure 3.17 Input voltage and output current for a capacitive force sensor. Capacitance is 1 pF and the ramp rate is 0.5 MV·s^{-1}

high capacitance. Polymeric foams that are made by dispersing a gas in a solid are ideal materials as they have good stability and low hysteresis.

Another method to measure the capacitance is to apply a triangular waveform (Figure 3.17).

$$v = \pm At \tag{3.27}$$

Differentiating

$$\frac{dv}{dt} = \pm A \tag{3.28}$$

Differentiating the voltage/current equation of a capacitor

$$C\frac{dv}{dt} = i \tag{3.29}$$

Eliminating dv/dt

$$i = \pm AC \tag{3.30}$$

The current is a square wave (Figure 3.17) and can be rectified producing an output that is constant for constant force (apart from the rapid transitions when the sign of the ramp changes). This method is sensitive to the small changes in capacitance for a sensor with a small surface area of less than 100 mm^2 that can be fitted to a fingertip or thumb. Figure 3.17 illustrates the values for a capacitance of 1 pF. Notice the small currents, but these can be detected with resistors and instrumentation amplifiers. A sensor for use in an artificial hand has been constructed that with a careful choice of foam material, separating the capacitor plates has a monotonic and repeatable characteristic [8].

3.2.5 Hall effect

Surface charges accumulate on a block of metal or semiconductor in the presence of a circulating current and magnetic field (Figure 3.18). The relationship between the charge carriers and magnetic field is

$$\boldsymbol{f} = q(\boldsymbol{v} \wedge \boldsymbol{B}) \tag{3.31}$$

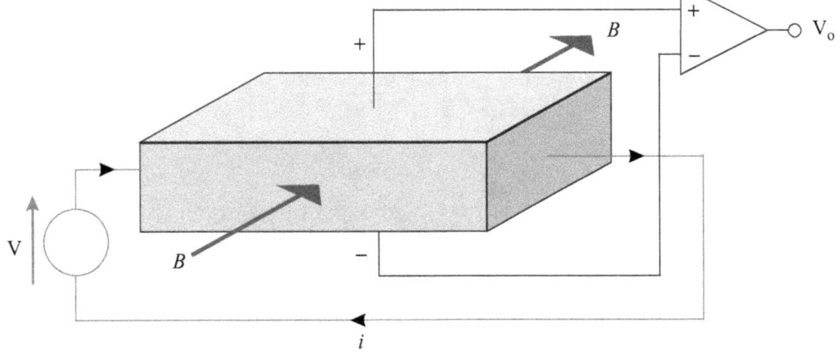

Figure 3.18 The Hall effect showing the applied voltage, V and magnetic field, B with an amplifier detecting the potential difference between the top and bottom surfaces of a semiconductor

where $\boldsymbol{f}$ is the magnetic force, q the charge on the carriers, $\boldsymbol{v}$ the average drift velocity and $\boldsymbol{B}$ the applied magnetic field. There is an accumulation of charge on the upper and lower surfaces as the carriers drift up or down. A balance occurs between the electric forces from the moving charges and magnetic forces resulting in a constant current, i, flowing across the material. An instrumentation amplifier is used to measure the potential difference across the block.

A force sensor can be made using this effect by varying the magnetic field, $\boldsymbol{B}$. Movement of a small magnet relative to the block alters the surface charge and the measured potential difference (Figure 3.18). An elastic material or spring relates the movement of the magnet to the applied force (Figure 3.19). Not shown in the figure is the housing to retain the components, which needs careful design. The spring and magnet are held in place with a circlip, e.g., so that they do not drop out of the housing when there is no force applied. A disadvantage of this method is the power consumption of the typical integrated circuit (IC) which can be several milliwatts. By suitable pulsing of the current or a sleep mode, the power consumption can be reduced but at the expense of additional components. Any external magnetic field will be sensed by the Hall effect IC and degrades the accuracy of the sensor. However, successful designs can be made that have good characteristics [9].

3.2.6 Quantum tunnelling composite

By combining the dielectric properties of a polymer material such as urethane or silicone with the conductive properties of a metal such as nickel, a quantum tunnelling composite (QTC) can be formed [10, 11]. This material has a high resistance at low forces and a low resistance at high forces with an approximately log-linear relationship. The resistance is almost open circuit to a few ohms with a high sensitivity at low forces. As a force sensor for artificial hands, some more development work is required to desensitise the low force performance, otherwise a QTC is only suitable for operation with small forces. Transient step changes in force produce slow recovery times that are not conducive to keeping a constant force in a closed-loop feedback system (from unrecorded experiments). Drift is also

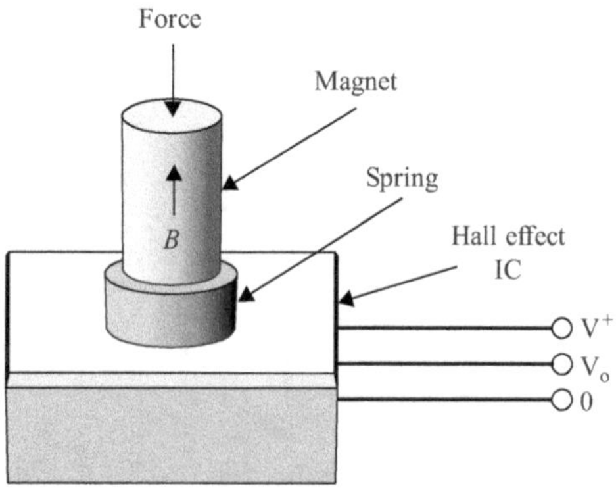

Figure 3.19 A Hall effect force sensor showing a magnet, spring and IC

present when a constant force is applied due to creep of the material. In its current form the sensitivity may be too high for use in an artificial hand [12].

3.3 Slip and texture sensors

3.3.1 Piezoelectric

The piezoelectric effect occurs in materials that when deformed produce a charge on the surface. Under no stress, a material has no overall electric charge (top side view of a square of the material is shown in Figure 3.20). On applying force in the

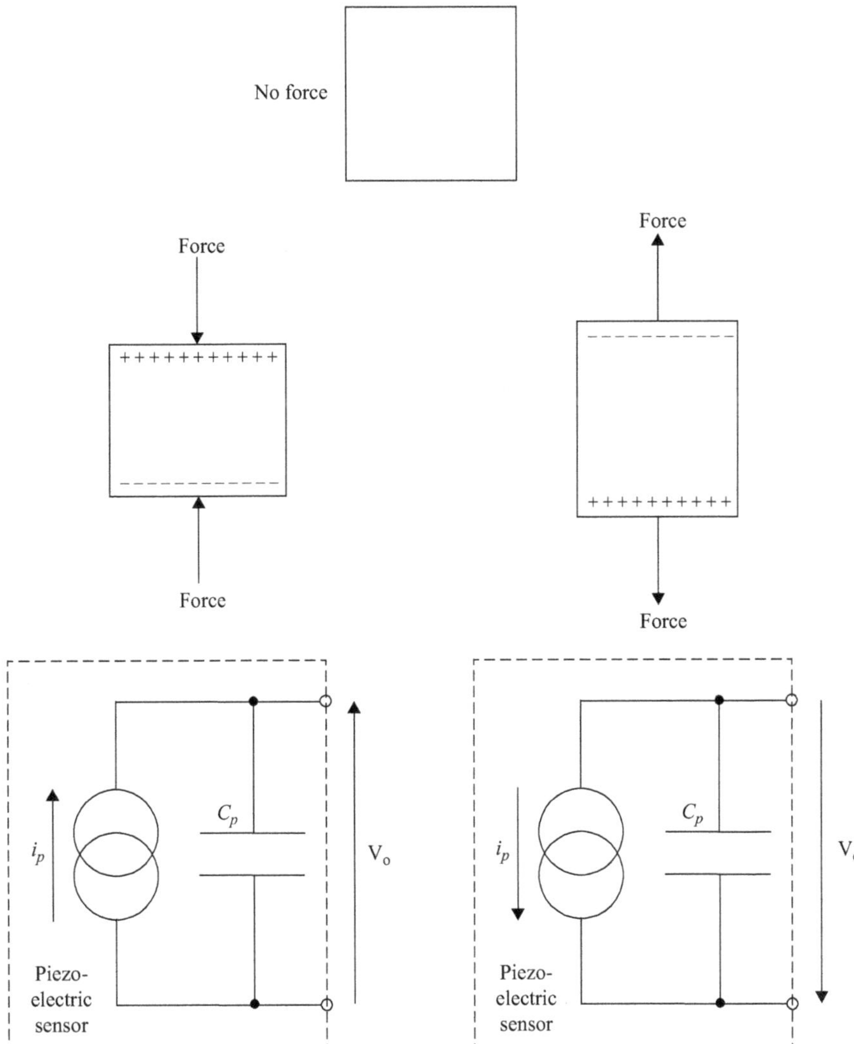

Figure 3.20 Illustration of a piezoelectric sensor

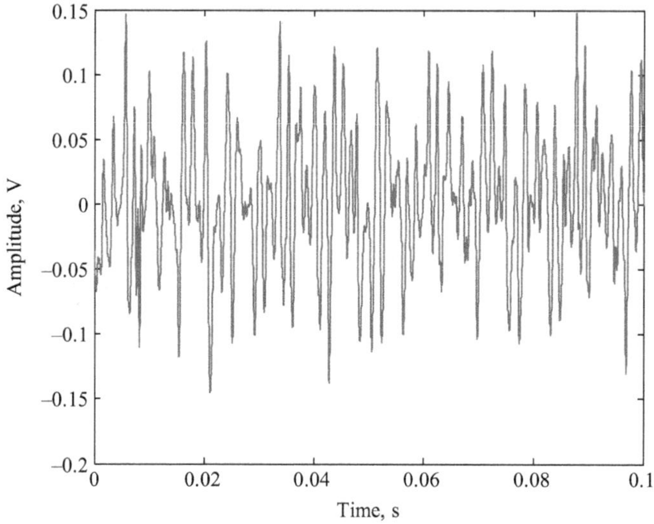

Figure 3.21 An example of the output signal from a fingertip sensor of the type shown in Figures 3.10 and 3.20 when the tip is passed at a constant velocity over a patterned surface

vertical direction to squash the material, positive charge is produced on the top with negative charge on the bottom (centre left in the figure). An equivalent electrical circuit for this effect is a current source in parallel with a capacitor (bottom left in the figure). Application of a force to elongate the material (middle right in the figure) creates the opposite charging effect. Consequently the polarity of the voltage reverses (lower right in the figure).

A typical piezoelectric sensor signal is shown in Figure 3.21. This output signal was obtained from the circuit shown in Figure 3.22, where there was a signal to noise ratio from the sensor system of 27dB (21 magnitude ratio). There was interference from the mains at 50 Hz, but this was only a peak value of 3 mV. However, there are repeating events in the signal, caused by a fingertip sensor (Figure 3.10) moving over a surface and detecting a repeating pattern of texture in the surface.

The charge from the sensor flows into the parallel combination of the sensor capacitance, C_p and the added resistance, R_a. There is a high frequency cut-off from this arrangement of

$$\omega = \frac{1}{(R_a C_p)} \tag{3.32}$$

The capacitance is typically 1 nF so if a cut-off of 1 kHz is required then from (3.32) the resistance, R_a, is

$$R_a = \frac{1}{2\pi f C_p} = \frac{1}{2\pi \times 10^3 \times 10^{-9}} = 159.15\,\text{k}\Omega \tag{3.33}$$

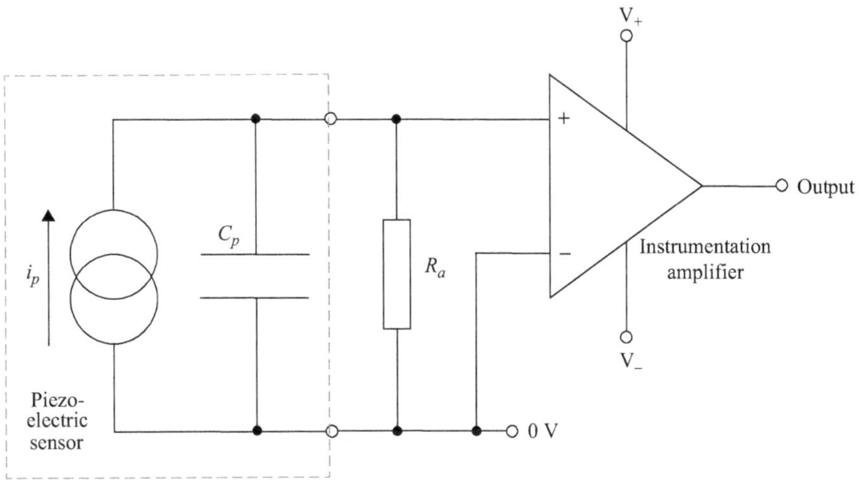

Figure 3.22 Piezoelectric sensor with instrumentation amplifier

However the current from the sensor is small and is typically 50 nA peak that corresponds to 7.9677 mV. Hence the amplifier should have a gain of about 100 corresponding to a signal magnitude of 0.79677 V. There is thus a trade-off between the desired frequency response and the gain of the instrumentation amplifier.

An alternative sensor circuit, using an operational amplifier, is shown in Figure 3.23. Here the charge from the piezoelectric material is integrated via the feedback capacitor, C_f. The feedback resistor, R_f, stabilises the circuit, otherwise the output drifts to one of the supply rails since the circuit will integrate any DC offset. The gain of the circuit is given by

$$G = \frac{C_p}{C_f} \tag{3.34}$$

To achieve a reasonable gain, the feedback capacitor, C_f, has a small value, but at the same time the frequency cut-off is determined by the choice of the feedback resistor, R_f which should be a large value.

The lower frequency cut-off is determined from the electromechanical characteristics of the sensor and is typically a few tens of hertz.

A standard method of analysing the data from a sensor is to use the Fast Fourier Transform (FFT) that shows the frequency content of a signal. As a simple example, consider Figure 3.24 that shows the FFT of a single sine wave, $y(t)$, with a frequency of 1 kHz and an amplitude of one. This plot is from a Matlab® program.

A new method to extract the frequency content of a signal uses the variance of the data. Originally the standard deviation was used but better sensitivity is achieved with the variance of the data. Unlike the FFT the method does not require selecting a suitable window to improve leakage (e.g., Hanning or Hamming), or padding the data set with additional zeroes for data lengths that are powers of two or the use of cosine and sine data in look-up tables. Instead the method involves the calculation of

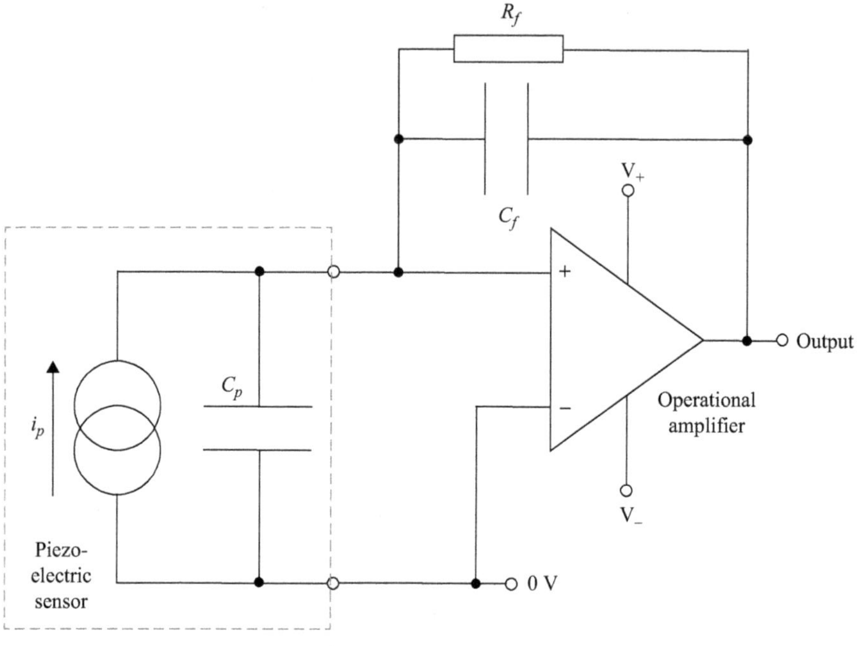

Figure 3.23 Piezoelectric sensor with operational amplifier

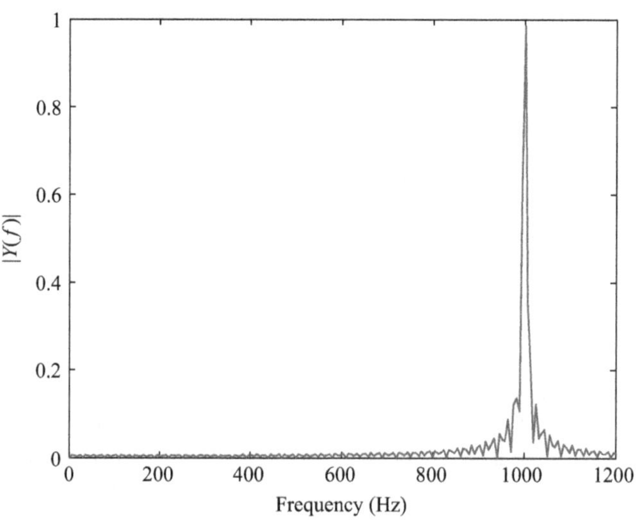

Figure 3.24 Single-sided amplitude spectrum of y(t) for a sine wave at 1 kHz

means of the data variance using simple arithmetic processes, i.e., simple additions, subtractions, divisions, multiplications and the summation of numbers.

Examples of the output from the new method are presented first together with the FFT analysis for comparison. The algorithm is presented later in the chapter.

Consider a sine wave of unity amplitude and at frequency of 1 kHz. The signal is sampled at 100 kHz (period 0.1 μs) and the data length is 10^5 samples (1 s). Figure 3.24 shows the results of the FFT analysis using Matlab® where as expected there is a peak at 1 kHz and some leakage. For the new method, Figure 3.25 shows the mean variance of the data plotted on the vertical axis against increasing window sizes of the data. At a window size of 100, there is a trough in the data that corresponds to a frequency of 1 kHz. This is calculated from the sampling frequency and window size, i.e., $10^5/100$. Therefore both the FFT and the new methods have correctly determined the frequency of the sine wave. The same averaged variance data can be replotted but with signal frequency shown on the horizontal axis (Figure 3.26). A further refinement is to rectify the averaged variance, and this is shown in Figure 3.27 by subtracting the mean variance of all the data, 0.5001, so that there is a peak shown in Figure 3.27 rather than the trough shown in Figure 3.26. The relationship between the peaks of rectified mean variance, meanvar, and the amplitude of a sine wave, A, is shown in Figure 3.28. The relationship is exactly as follows.

$$A = \sqrt{2\,\text{meanvar}} \tag{3.35}$$

The algorithm consists of putting the data (n samples) into windows, calculating the variance using successive data samples in each window and then taking the average of the variances.

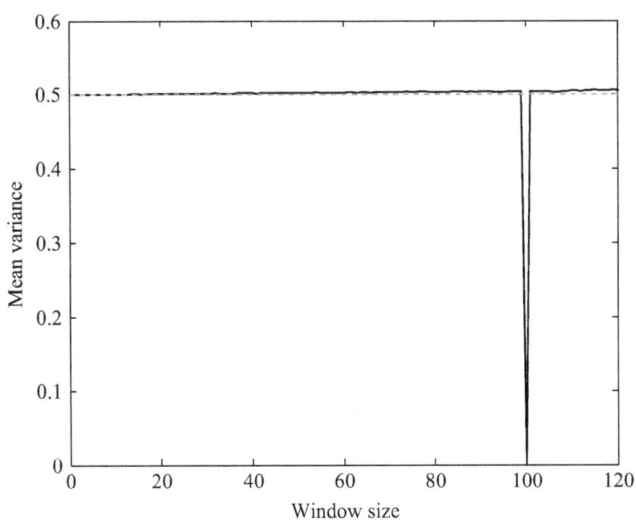

Figure 3.25 Mean variance plotted against window size of y(t) for a sine wave at 1 kHz. The horizontal line at 0.5001 is the variance of all the data

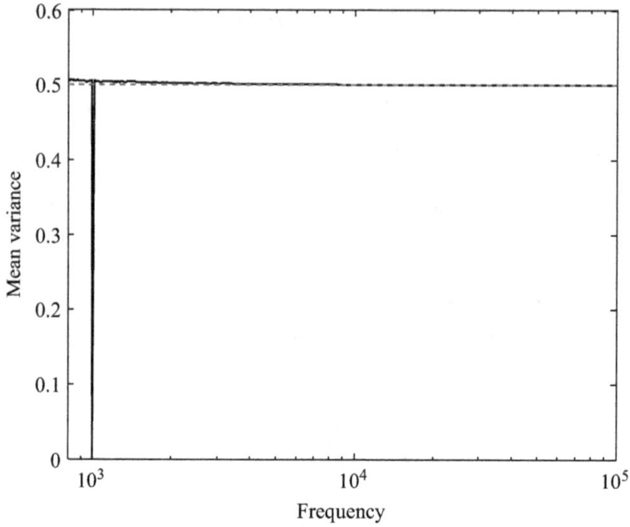

Figure 3.26 *Mean variance plotted against frequency for a sine wave at 1 kHz. The horizontal line at 0.5001 is the variance of all the data*

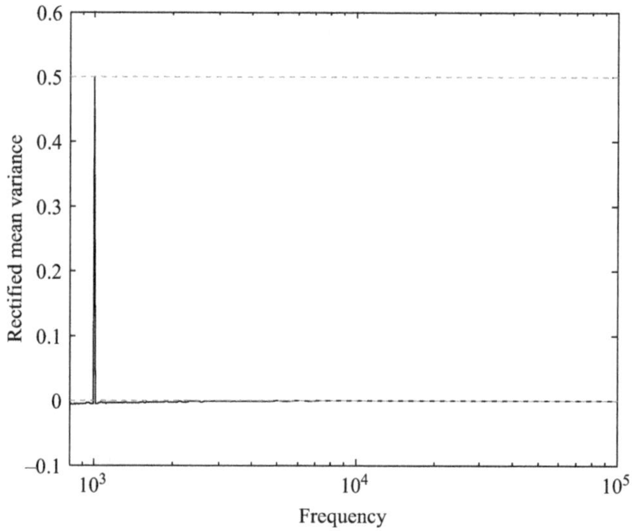

Figure 3.27 *Rectified mean variance plotted against frequency for a sine wave at 1 kHz. The horizontal line at 0.5001 is the variance of all the data*

The variance, var, is

$$\text{var} = \frac{1}{n-1}\sum_{j=1}^{n}\left(d_j - \bar{d}\right)^2 \tag{3.36}$$

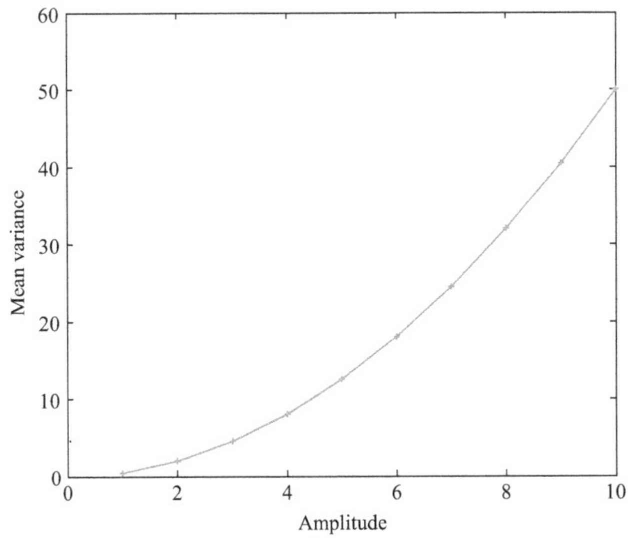

Figure 3.28 Peaks of rectified mean variance against amplitude

where the mean is

$$\bar{d} = \frac{1}{n}\sum_{j=1}^{n} d_j \tag{3.37}$$

The data is divided into windows of length W. These window lengths are ranged over the data such that

$$\text{var}_i = \text{var}\left(d_i, d_{i+w}, \ldots d_{i+(M-1)W}\right) \tag{3.38}$$

$$\text{meanvar} = \text{mean}(\text{var}_1, \text{var}_2, \ldots, \text{var}_M) \tag{3.39}$$

where

The sampled data is

$$d = d_1, d_2, \ldots, d_n \tag{3.40}$$

The windows are ranged over i

$$i = 1, 2, \ldots, W \tag{3.41}$$

The number of windows is ranged over m

$$m = 1, 2, \ldots, M \tag{3.42}$$

An example set of data that are random numbers, with a uniform distribution in the range (-1 to 1) is shown in Figure 3.29 where the calculation is made for the first 20 samples ($n = 20$). The illustration is for the window length of five ($W = 5$) and there are thus four windows ($M = 4$). The first variance of data is calculated

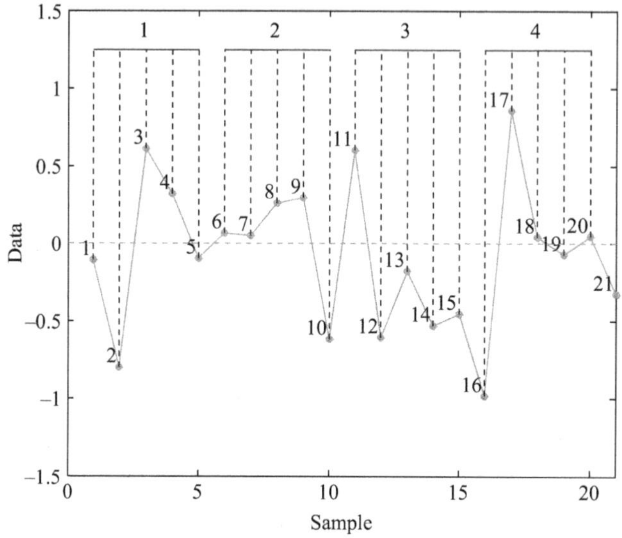

Figure 3.29 An example of the calculation for a random uniform set of data. There are four windows (M = 4) and the length of each window is five (W = 5) for the data set of n = 20

from the first sample in each window and then the second sample in each window and so on.

$$\mathrm{var}_1 = \mathrm{var}(d_1, d_6, d_{11}, d_{16}) \tag{3.43}$$

$$\mathrm{var}_2 = \mathrm{var}(d_2, d_7, d_{12}, d_{17}) \tag{3.44}$$

$$\mathrm{var}_3 = \mathrm{var}(d_3, d_8, d_{13}, d_{18}) \tag{3.45}$$

$$\mathrm{var}_4 = \mathrm{var}(d_4, d_9, d_{14}, d_{19}) \tag{3.46}$$

$$\mathrm{var}_5 = \mathrm{var}(d_5, d_{10}, d_{15}, d_{20}) \tag{3.47}$$

The mean variance is the mean of all the variances and is simply

$$\mathrm{meanvar} = \mathrm{mean}(\mathrm{var}_1, \mathrm{var}_2, \mathrm{var}_3, \mathrm{var}_4, \mathrm{var}_5) \tag{3.48}$$

The illustration is for four windows ($M = 4$) and the length of each window is five (W = 5) as shown in Table 3.2, so there are five variances to be calculated. Since the number of windows and their lengths are integers, then not all the samples can be included in all the calculations. The example over states this exclusion of samples in that the number of data samples is small compared to the practical use where thousands or more samples are used. In practice, the loss of a small number of samples has little impact on the method results.

A sensor, moved across a machined surface that has a repeating pattern, such as a series of grooved lines, will have a signal with repeating characteristics.

Table 3.2 Data and windows for the example in Figure 3.29

M	W	d_1	d_2	d_3	d_4	d_5	d_6	d_7	d_8	d_9	d_{10}	d_{11}	d_{12}	d_{13}	d_{14}	d_{15}	d_{16}	d_{17}	d_{18}	d_{19}	d_{20}
1	20	a	b	c	d	e	f	g	h	i	j	k	l	m	n	o	p	q	r	s	t
2	10	a	b	c	d	e	f	g	h	i	j	a	b	c	d	e	f	g	h	i	j
3	6	a	b	c	d	e	f	a	b	c	d	e	f	a	b	c	d	e	f		
4	5	a	b	c	d	e	a	b	c	d	e	a	b	c	d	e	a	b	c	d	e
5	4	a	b	c	d	a	b	c	d	a	b	c	d	a	b	c	d	a	b	c	d
6	3	a	b	c	a	b	c	a	b	c	a	b	c	a	b	c	a	b	c		
7	2	a	b	a	b	a	b	a	b	a	b	a	b	a	b						
8	2	a	b	a	b	a	b	a	b	a	b	a	b	a	b	a	b				
9	2	a	b	a	b	a	b	a	b	a	b	a	b	a	b	a	b	a	b		
10	2	a	b	a	b	a	b	a	b	a	b	a	b	a	b	a	b	a	b	a	b
11	1	a	a	a	a	a	a	a	a	a	a	a									
12	1	a	a	a	a	a	a	a	a	a	a	a	a								
13	1	a	a	a	a	a	a	a	a	a	a	a	a	a							
14	1	a	a	a	a	a	a	a	a	a	a	a	a	a	a						
15	1	a	a	a	a	a	a	a	a	a	a	a	a	a	a	a					
16	1	a	a	a	a	a	a	a	a	a	a	a	a	a	a	a	a				
17	1	a	a	a	a	a	a	a	a	a	a	a	a	a	a	a	a	a			
18	1	a	a	a	a	a	a	a	a	a	a	a	a	a	a	a	a	a	a		
19	1	a	a	a	a	a	a	a	a	a	a	a	a	a	a	a	a	a	a	a	
20	1	a	a	a	a	a	a	a	a	a	a	a	a	a	a	a	a	a	a	a	a

In each row, the letters refer to the data samples for each variance calculation. On the row where $M = 4$ and $W = 5$ the 'a's form the first calculation of variance (6.9), the 'b's the second calculation (6.10), etc.

The dimension of the surface pattern, d; the relative velocity, v, of the surface moving with respect to the sensor; the window size, W, and sampling frequency, f, are related. For a large dimension of the pattern, there will be a low-frequency component for a low velocity when the sensor is moved across a textured surface. Increasing the velocity will increase the frequency of the output signal. For a given velocity, if the dimension of the pattern is small then the sensor signal will have a higher frequency component compared to a larger dimension in the pattern.

The sampling frequency for n samples taken over a time, t, is

$$f = \frac{n}{t} \tag{3.49}$$

The dimension and velocity are related by

$$v = \frac{d}{t} = df \tag{3.50}$$

For a given dimension

$$n > \frac{df}{v} \quad \text{or} \quad W > \frac{df}{v} \tag{3.51}$$

Figure 3.30 shows the voltage output from an amplifier connected to a piezoelectric sensor mounted on a fingertip when it is passed by a pattern that has repeating notches scored every 0.2 mm. The surface has a repeating pattern as shown in Figure 3.31. The test acrylic strip is attached to an aluminium tube and then moved past the fingertip (Figure 3.32). In between the fingertip surface and test strip

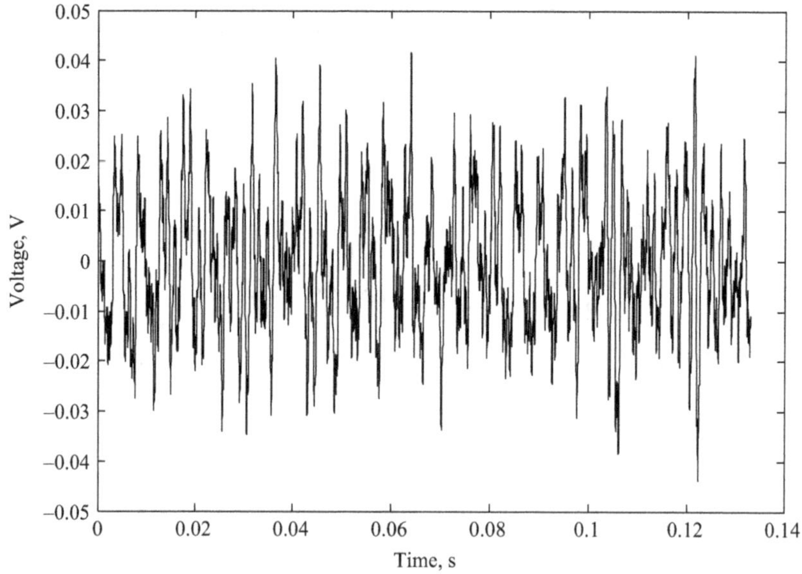

Figure 3.30 Piezoelectric signal

is a piece of silicone glove. The position of the textured surface relative to the sensor was measured with a digital slotted-opto sensor (Figure 3.33). From these data, knowing the separation of the slots, the velocity of the surface is calculated (Figure 3.34). The velocity is fairly constant and has a mean value of 46.9 mm·s^{-1}.

In Figure 3.35 the first minima (notch) occurs at 0.004482 s. The dimension, d, from (6.16) is

$$d = vt = 0.2102 \text{ mm} \tag{3.52}$$

The calculated value is 5% different from the average measured grating dimension using a microscope of 0.2 mm. The mean variance can be plotted against frequency (Figures 3.36 and 3.37).

The dimension of the grating can also be calculated from the FFT of the piezoelectric signal (Figure 3.38). The dominant peak in the plot occurs at 220.3 Hz.

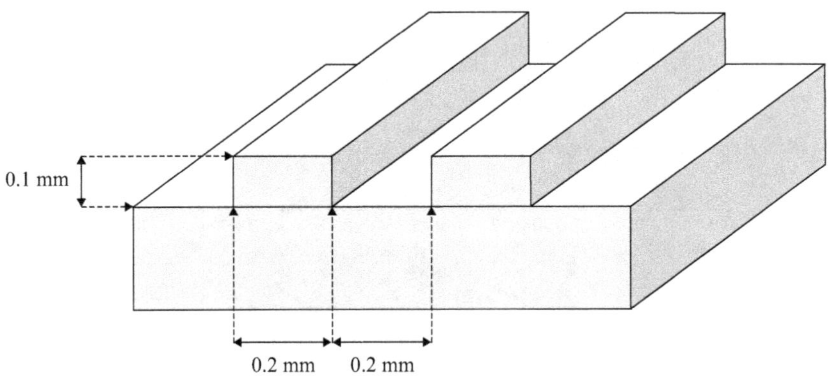

Figure 3.31 Textured surface on acrylic test strip

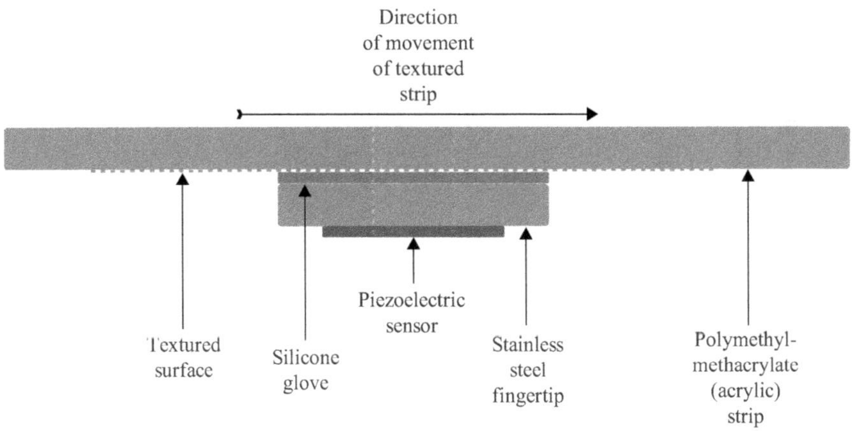

Figure 3.32 Diagrammatic top view of textured surface and fingertip with a piezoelectric sensor

Hence the dimension is

$$d = \frac{v}{f} = \frac{46.9}{220.3} = 0.2129 \text{ mm} \tag{3.53}$$

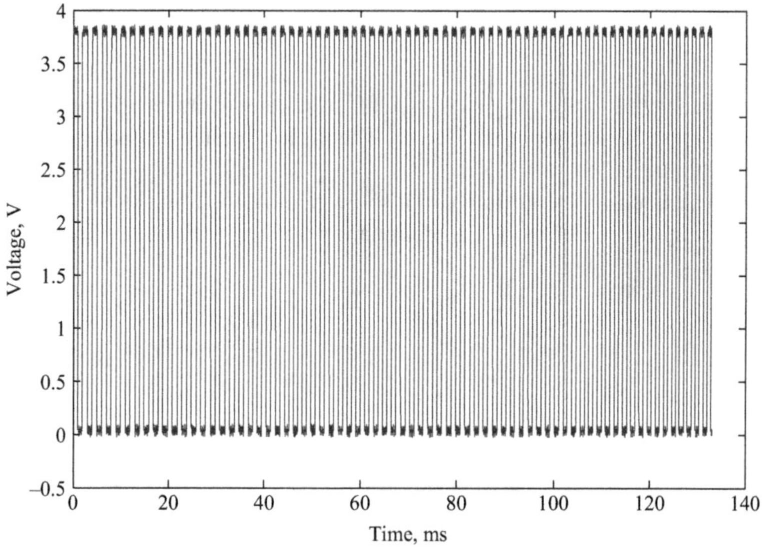

Figure 3.33 Encoder digital signal

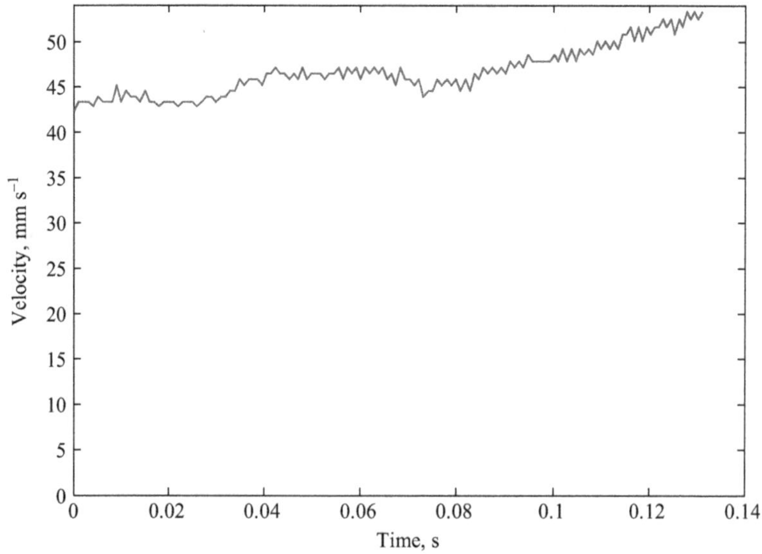

Figure 3.34 Velocity of the tube and textured surface

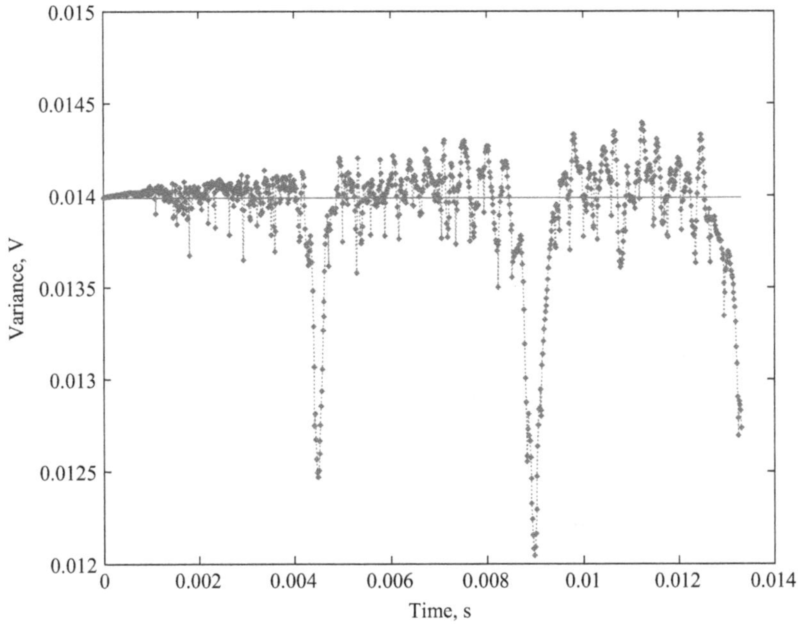

Figure 3.35 Mean variance against time. Horizontal line shows the variance of all the data

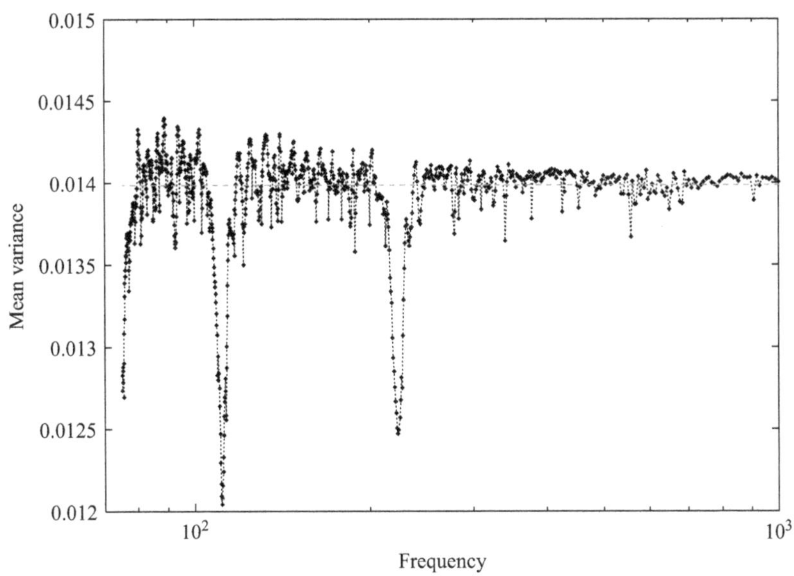

Figure 3.36 Mean variance against frequency. Horizontal line shows the variance of all the data

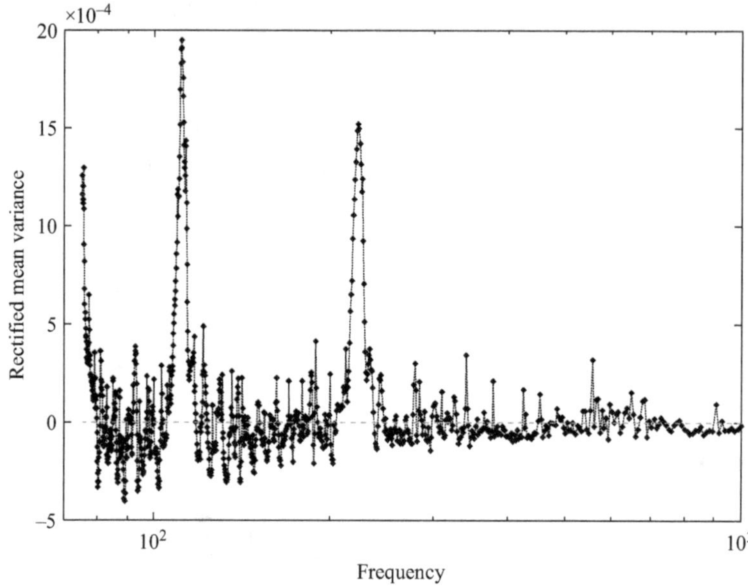

Figure 3.37 Rectified mean variance

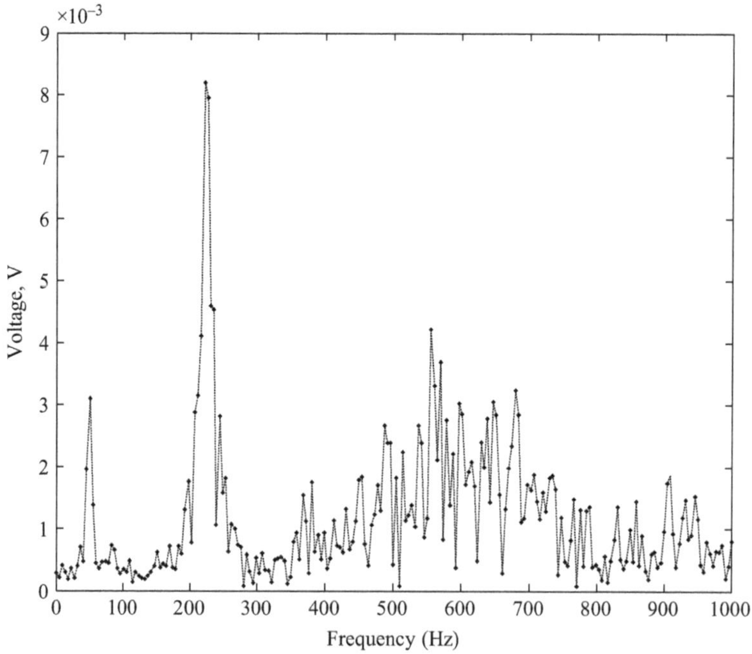

Figure 3.38 FFT of the data

The calculated value is 6.5% different from the average measured grating dimension using a microscope of 0.2 mm.

The second minima occurs at 0.008977 s which is twice the time for the first minima (0.008977/0.004482 = 2.003 s). There are further minima at multiples of the first minima. This effect is not surprising as the method is detecting signal values that have the same values at repeating instances in time. Further investigation is required to see if this information can be used in an algorithm that makes the detection of frequencies more robust from the variance plot. Maxima and minima can be determined automatically by setting thresholds and boundaries using, e.g., 'findpeaks' in Matlab®.

An experiment conducted at a higher mean velocity of 98.5 mm·s^{-1} produced similar results for the estimate of the spacing of the grating of the textured surface. Figure 3.39 shows the signal and Figure 3.40 the velocity. From the variance analysis there is a peak at 482 Hz (Figure 3.41), and from the FFT a peak at 481.9 Hz (Figure 3.42) from which the distance is calculated as 0.205 mm. However, if the velocity varies as shown in Figures 3.43 and 3.44, there is a range of the frequencies (Figures 3.45 and 3.46). The mean velocity is 51.9 mm·s^{-1} in a range from about 35 to 70 mm·s^{-1}. There are peaks in the variance and FFT plots at 525.8 and 523.2 Hz, respectively, and the distances calculated from these values are 0.0987 and 0.0992 mm, respectively. These values are approximately half the actual dimension of 0.2 mm. It is therefore important to maintain a constant velocity while gathering data from the sensor.

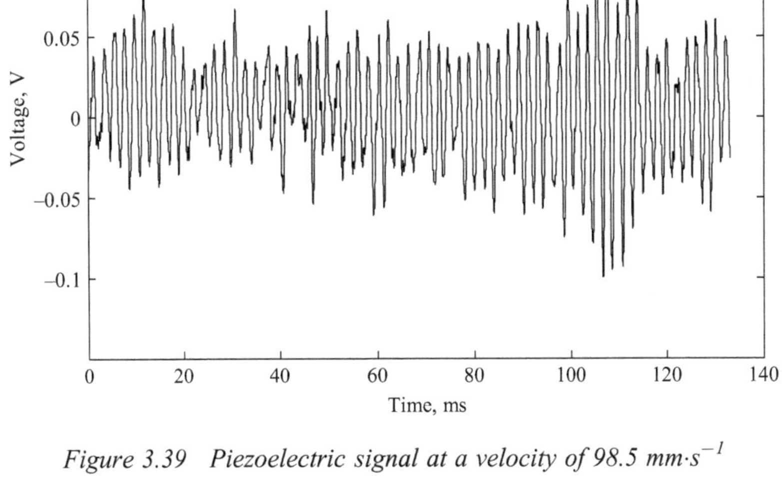

Figure 3.39 Piezoelectric signal at a velocity of 98.5 mm·s^{-1}

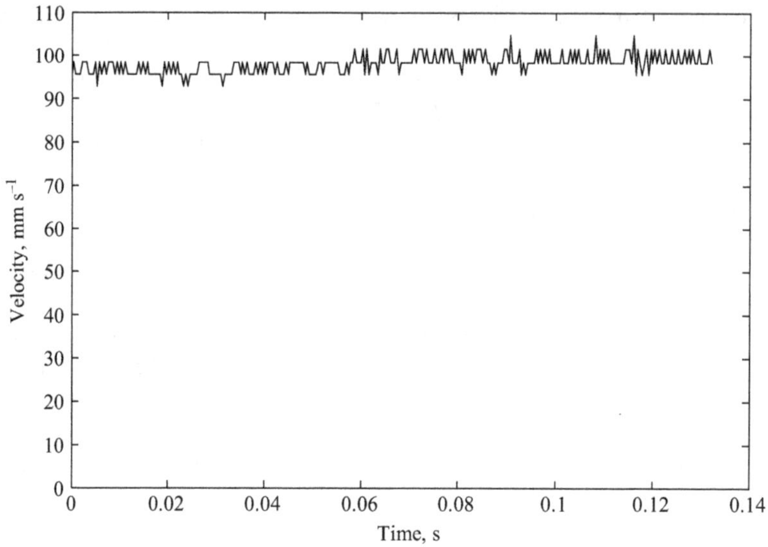

Figure 3.40 Velocity of the tube and textured surface at a mean velocity of 98.5 mm·s^{-1}

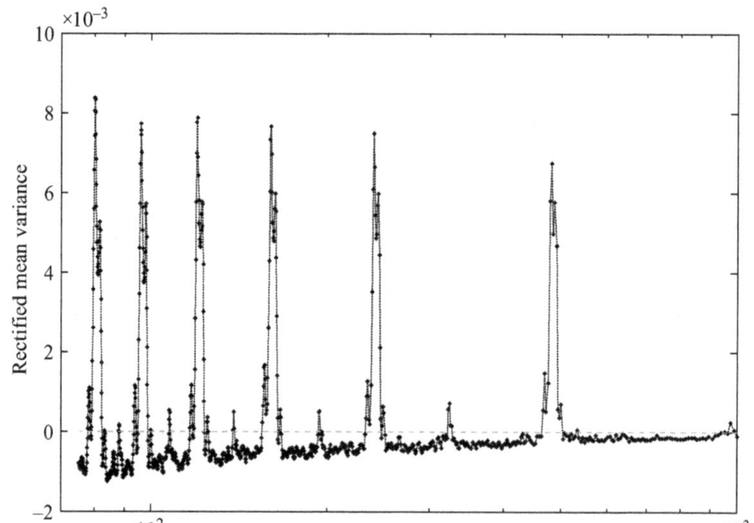

Figure 3.41 Rectified mean variance for a mean velocity of 98.5 mm·s^{-1}

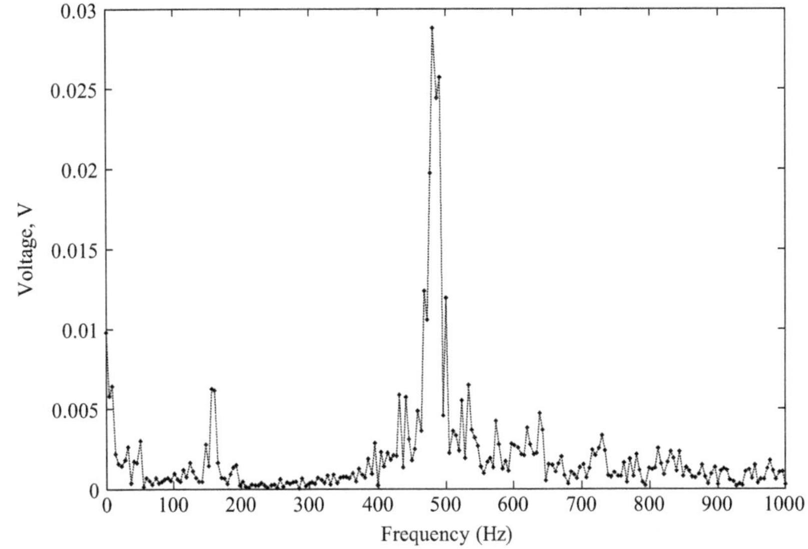

Figure 3.42 FFT at a mean velocity of 98.5 mm·s^{-1}

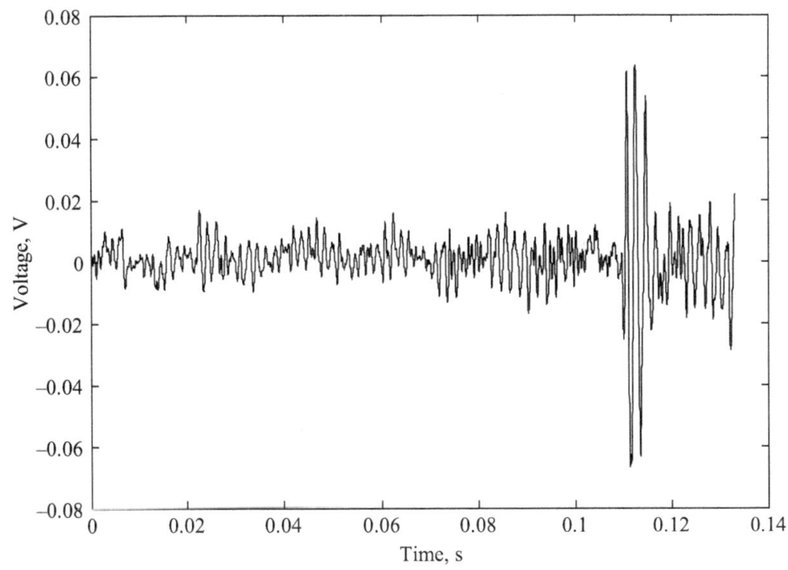

Figure 3.43 Piezoelectric signal in a velocity range from 35 to 70 mm·s^{-1}

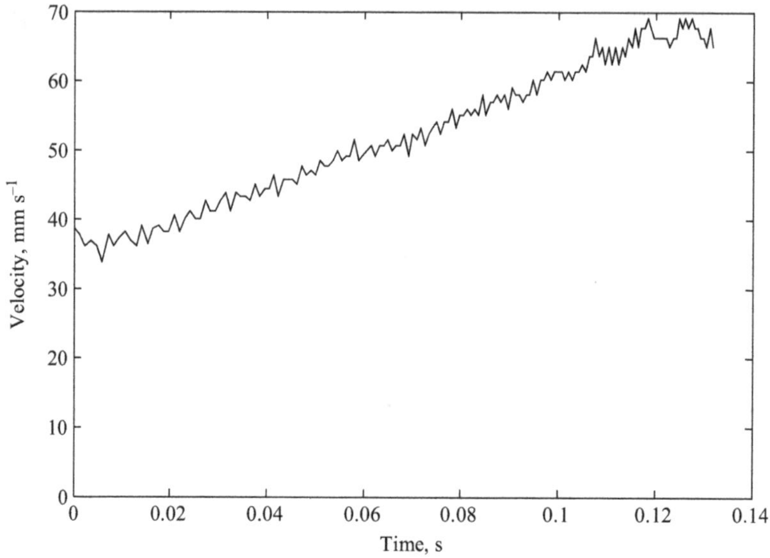

Figure 3.44 Velocity ramp in a velocity range from 35 to 70 mm·s^{-1}

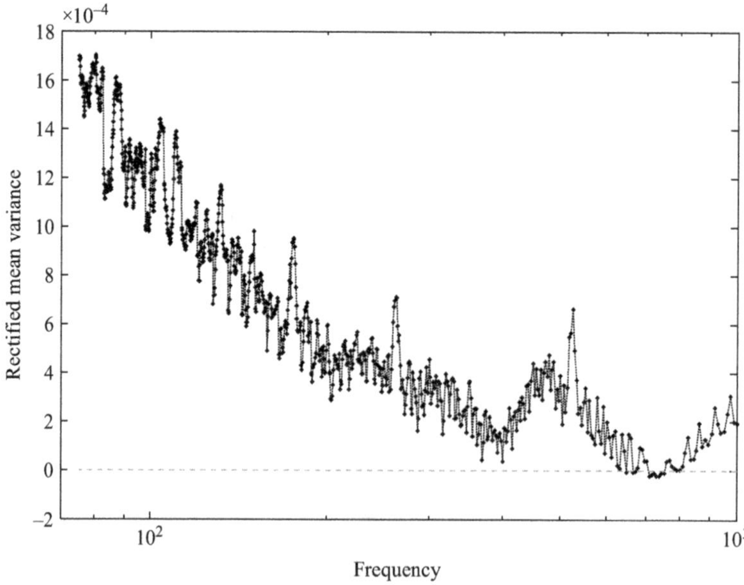

Figure 3.45 Rectified mean variance in a velocity range from 35 to 70 mm·s^{-1}

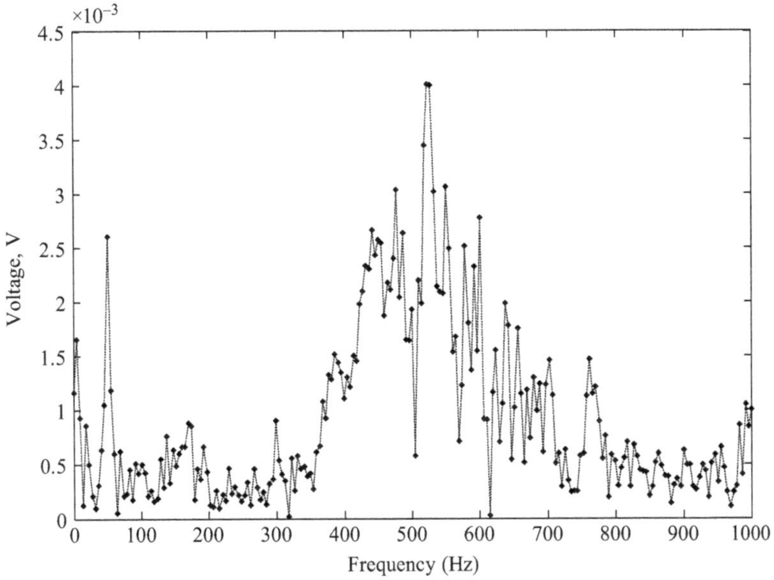

Figure 3.46 FFT in a velocity range from 35 to 70 mm·s^{-1}

3.3.2 Roller ball using a wheel to detect slip

If a wheel or sphere is in contact with an object, then any rotation can be detected by an optical encoder. However, most prosthetic hands are covered by a glove that will cover any sensors. Object slip will therefore not be detected, and a roller ball is not a practical method.

3.3.3 Acoustic

Acoustic noise generated between the surface of an object and a fingertip can be detected with a miniature microphone. These microphones are used in hearing aids. Slip detection can be combined with force measurement using an optical method (Section 3.4.3). To combat sounds from other sources, a second microphone should be mounted in the hand and any common mode signals can then be removed. The microphones have to be mechanically integrated into the structure of a hand, as they are not thin so they do not lie flat on the surface of a fingertip.

3.3.4 Arrays of force sensors

Movement of the natural hand and fingers is achieved by combining information from sensors in joints, muscles, skin and tendons. Object grip is maintained by the information from these sensors that is feedback to the neural system. Similarly, object movement in an artificial hand can also be coordinated by combining information from a number of sensors. Consider four force sensors mounted close together (Figure 3.47) at a fingertip. Movement of a held object may result in magnitude

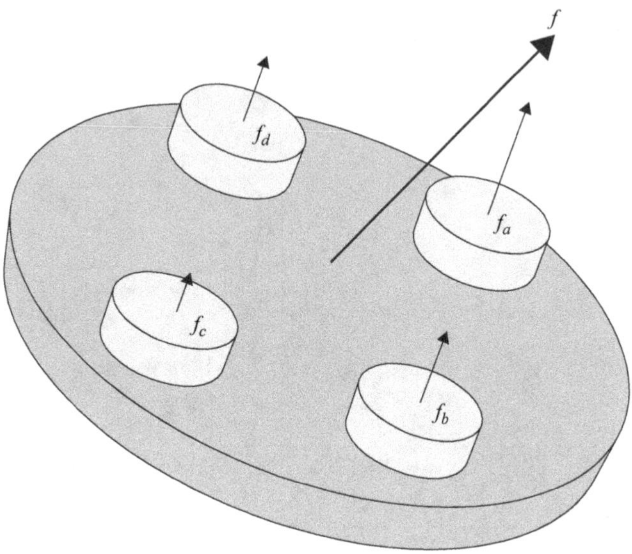

*Figure 3.47 The sensing of four normal forces, f_a, f_b, f_c, and f_d are combined into one force vector, **f**. Any changes in **f** estimates the slip direction of a held object*

changes and direction changes of a resultant force formed by combining the normal forces from the sensors, thereby giving an estimation of the direction of slip [13, 14].

3.3.5 Accelerometer

Micro-electro-mechanical systems (MEMS) in the form of accelerometers detect the acceleration of a body in one, two or three directions. These devices can output a signal when they sense the relative movement between a finger and an object. Accelerometers are small, low-cost and low-power devices that are suitable for application to artificial hands. However, accelerometers sense both linear acceleration and that is due to the Earth's gravitational field. An accelerometer in a moving hand experiences changes due to linear acceleration and orientation with respect to the Earth's field. Careful signal processing is required to estimate the slip signal. One possible method is to high pass filter the signal. An accelerometer moving in the x direction on a flat horizontal surface is orthogonal to the direction of the Earth's field and is therefore not influenced by the acceleration due to gravity (Figure 3.48). The output signal, s, from the accelerometer is

$$s = \ddot{x} \tag{3.54}$$

where $\ddot{x}$ is the acceleration in the x direction.

Consider the accelerometer moving in the x-z plane only (Figure 3.49) where it accelerates away from the flat surface at an angle, θ. The output signal is

$$s = \ddot{x} \cos\theta \tag{3.55}$$

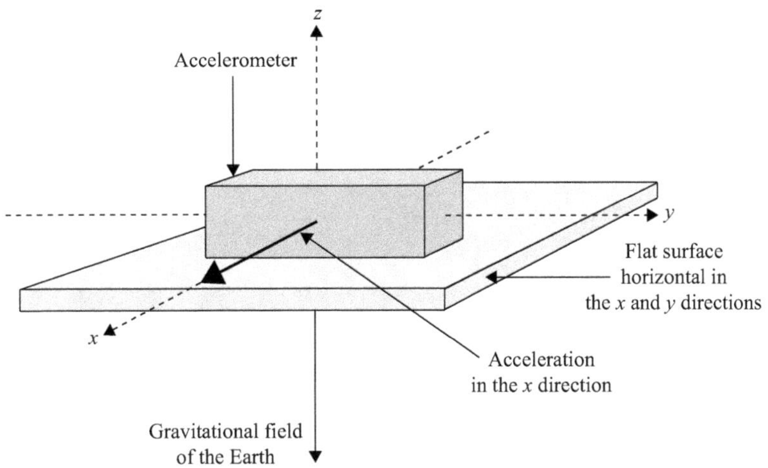

Figure 3.48 An accelerometer on a flat surface accelerated in the x direction

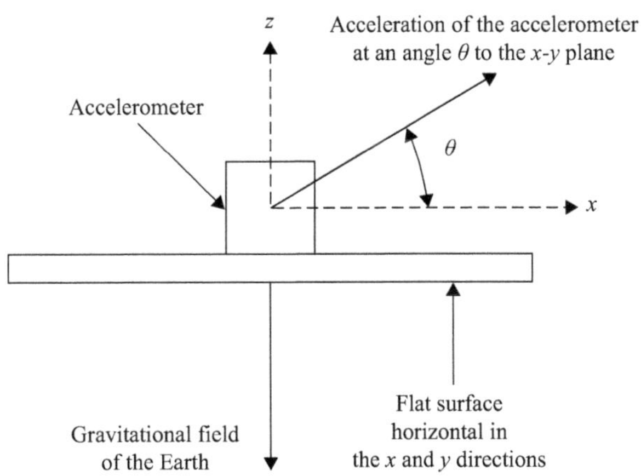

Figure 3.49 An accelerometer accelerated in the x-z plane in a direction at an angle θ

If the accelerometer is inclined at an angle, θ, to the x-z plane (Figures 3.50 and 3.51) and is not moving then

$$s = g\cos\theta \tag{3.56}$$

Maintaining the inclination of the accelerometer and accelerating in the x direction, then

$$s = \ddot{x}\cos\theta + g\cos\theta \tag{3.57}$$

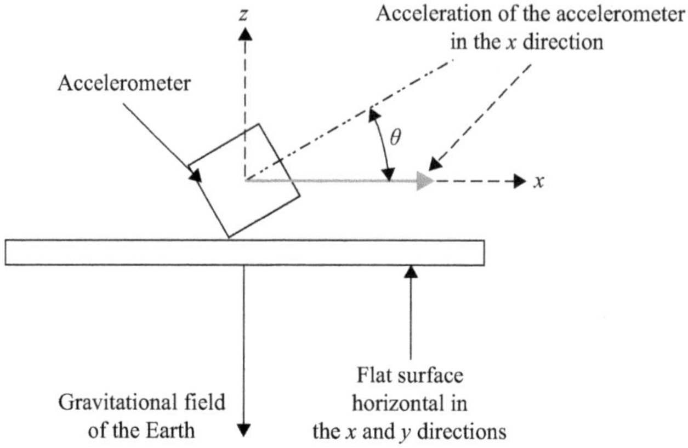

Figure 3.50 Acceleration in the x direction while inclined at an angle θ

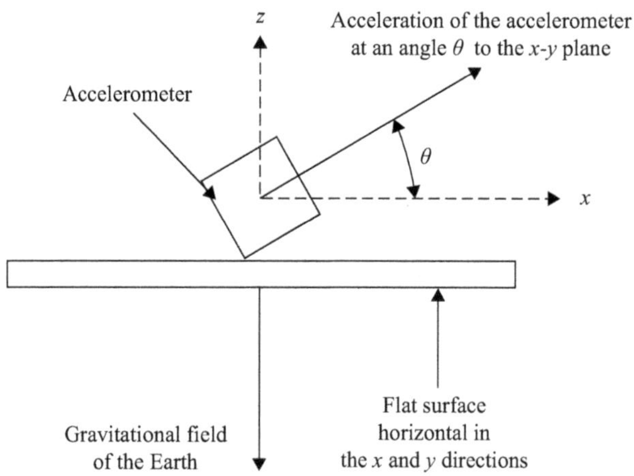

Figure 3.51 Acceleration of an accelerometer inclined at an angle, θ, to the horizontal

Upon accelerating at an angle, θ, away from the flat surface, the output signal is

$$s = \ddot{x} + g\cos\theta \tag{3.58}$$

For a single axis accelerometer, it's orientation in the x-z plane has an effect on the gravitational component that is a cosine function of the angle made with respect to the Earth's gravitational field. It's inclination to the x-axis and direction of movement also influences the output signal.

However, more typically, an accelerometer is subjected to accelerations in all three directions. Furthermore, a three-axis accelerometer has three orthogonally placed accelerometers with a coordinate frame x_a, y_a and z_a (Figure 3.52).

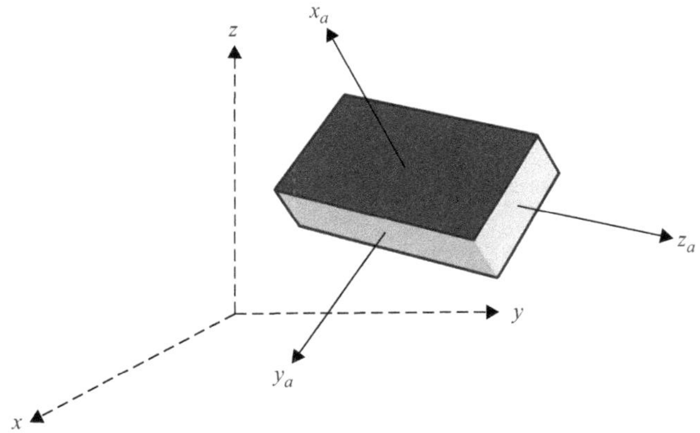

Figure 3.52 A three-dimensional accelerometer with axes x_a, y_a and z_a orientated to an Earth reference frame x, y, z

The accelerometer package is oriented with respect to an Earth reference frame, x, y and z. Equations for all three accelerometers can be formed

$$s_a = f_a(\theta, \beta, \gamma, \ddot{x}, \ddot{y}, \ddot{z}) \tag{3.59}$$

$$s_b = f_b(\theta, \beta, \gamma, \ddot{x}, \ddot{y}, \ddot{z}) \tag{3.60}$$

$$s_c = f_c(\theta, \beta, \gamma, \ddot{x}, \ddot{y}, \ddot{z}) \tag{3.61}$$

where θ, β and γ are the angles of the three-axis accelerometer with respect to the x-z, x-y and z-y planes. The output signals are s_a, s_b and s_c. To extract the three accelerations requires estimates of the three angles that can be from MEMS rate gyros. It can be seen from the complexity of these system equations that the estimation of a slip signal in practice is not simple.

An artificial hand using signals from a set of MEMS devices could estimate its orientation and would be useful in the operation of a whole arm where there are elbow and shoulder joints.

3.4 Position (angle)

The design of the mechanical links in a finger produces a defined curling action, so that the tip of the finger can be determined analytically from a measurement of the angle of the joint at the finger base (metacarpal joint). A sensor mounted at this joint can then be used in a closed-loop positioning system. It is also possible to sense position further back in the mechanism, i.e., in the gearbox. Where a linear actuator is used, the technologies for rotatory sensors are also applicable to linear sensors.

3.4.1 Rotary potentiometer

Miniature potentiometers are simple and low-cost components that provide a potential divider where the output voltage is proportional to angle of the shaft. However,

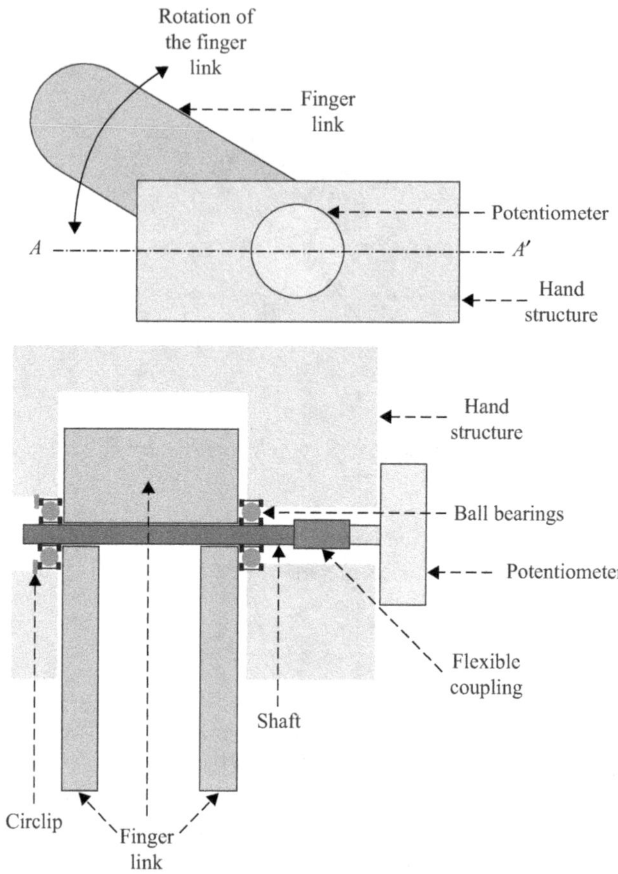

Figure 3.53 Diagrammatic assembly of a finger base joint. The top drawing shows a side view. The lower drawing shows top view of a cross-section AA′

connecting a shaft of a potentiometer to a finger joint can be problematic. A potentiometer has a shaft and body where the resistance element is housed. The body is attached to the hand structure either with adhesive, clamps or bolts, which is simple but the centre axis of the shaft should be aligned with that of the axle of the lowest finger link (Figure 3.53). This is unlikely to happen in practice since the sizes of the structures are small and potentiometers are not generally made accurately for position measurements. To overcome this problem a small flexible coupling can connect the potentiometer shaft to that of the finger to mitigate any misalignment of the two shafts. A further disadvantage of this method is that the potentiometer housing protrudes at the edge of the hand structure and there may not be enough space to accommodate a potentiometer at the sides of the middle and third fingers. The rotation of lower finger link is less than 90 degrees so only one-third of the potential 270-degree range may be used reducing the performance of a potentiometer.

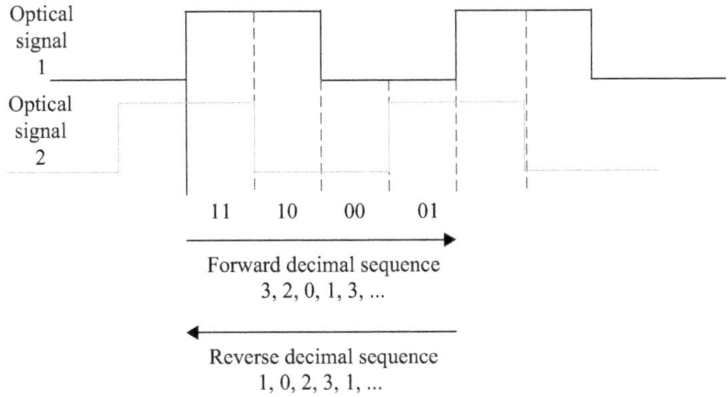

Figure 3.54 Complementary binary pair of signals showing the two sequences of forward and reverse rotation of an optical encoder

3.4.2 Hall effect

A small magnet attached to the shaft of a lower link in a finger can be sensed by a Hall effect IC with good linearity and accuracy. A small IC can be mounted on the hand structure making a good solution to the measurement of finger position. An advantage of this method is that it is non-contact. However, it has the same disadvantages of force measurement, i.e., the circuits have high power consumption and the devices are susceptible to interference from stray environmental magnetic fields.

3.4.3 Optics

A compact solution to sensing the fingertip position is to use an optical encoder mounted on the back of a motor or gearbox. There are two complementary output signals from a typical encoder, so that the direction of rotation can be sensed but not the absolute positon (Figure 3.54). On applying power to a hand, the fingers must first be moved to an end position either fully flexed into the palm or fully extended to form a flat hand. Some encoders provide a third channel for synchronisation once every revolution. As there is usually a reduction gearbox in transmission mechanism, a modest resolution encoder produces a high-resolution measurement. A disadvantage of this method is that no account is taken of backlash in the finger links or transmission mechanism. An optical encoder is a high-cost solution to position measurement but is compact if the motor is mounted in the palm; the interconnecting wires do not experience any fatigue if they are flexed round a finger joint.

3.5 Summary

Signals from sensors are used in closed-loop feedback systems to automatically adjust variables such as grip force to arrest object slip. Also information from sensors can also be used to alert the wearer of a hand that an object is too hot to hold, for example. Resistive, capacitive, inductive, optical and Hall effect technologies can all be used to form sensors. Sensors can be made of low-cost and low-power technologies from screen printable piezoresistive and piezoelectric materials, which are used to measure forces in the fingers and thumb and to detect slip or surface texture. Analogue electronics in the form of instrumentation amplifiers condition the signal from a sensor. Digital processing of the analogue signal from a texture sensor mounted on a fingertip reveals the repeating pattern and coarseness of an object surface. A novel form of signal processing, using the rectified mean variance of the signal (equivalent to the FFT) is used in this analysis.

References

1 Cotton D. P. J, Cranny A., White N. M., Chappell P. H., and Beeby S. P. 'A novel thick-film piezoelectric slip sensor for a prosthetic hand', *IEEE Sensors Journal: Special Edition on Intelligent Sensors*, 2007;**7**(5):752–761

2 Cranny A, Cotton D. P. J., Chappell P. H., Beeby S. P., and White N. M. 'Thick-film force and slip sensors for a prosthetic hand, *Sensors and Actuators A: Physical*, 2005;**123–124**:162–171

3 Cranny A., Cotton D. P. J., Chappell P. H., Beeby S. P., and White N. M. 'Thick-film force and slip sensors for a prosthetic hand', *Measurement Science and Technology*, 2005;**16**:931–941

4 Cotton D. P. J., Cranny A., Chappell P. H., and White N. M. 'Thick-film piezoelectric slip sensors for automatic grip control in prosthetic hands', *12th World Congress International Society of Prosthetics and Orthotics*, Vancouver, Canada, 2007, 4

5 Muridan N., Chappell P. H., Cotton D. P. J., Cranny A., and White N. M. 'Detection of slip from multiple sites in an artificial finger', *Sensors & Their Applications XV*, IOP ISSN 1742-6588, Edinburgh Scotland, 2009, 1–6

6 Chappell P. H., Cotton D. P. J. Cranny A., and White N. M. 'Experimental lead zirconate titanate (PZT) slip sensor', *MEC' 08*, University of New Brunswick, Fredericton, Canada, 2008, 204–207

7 Kyberd P. J. and Chappell P. H. 'Characterization of an optical and acoustic touch and slip sensor for autonomous manipulation', *Measurement Science and Technology*, 1992;**3**:969–975

8 Chappell P. H. and Elliott J. A. 'Contact force sensor for artificial hands with a digital interface for a controller', *Measurement Science and Technology*, 2003;**14**:1275–1279

9 Kyberd P. J. and Chappell P. H. 'A force sensor for automatic manipulation based on the Hall effect', *Measurement Science and Technology*, 1993;**4**:281–287

10 Bloor D., Donnelly K., Hands P. J., Laughin P., and Lussey D. 'A metal-polymer composite with unusual properties', *Journal Physics D Applied Physics*, 2005;**38**:2851–2860

11 Bloor D., Graham A., Williams E. J., Laughin P., and Lussey D. 'Metal-polymer composite with nanostructure filler particles and amplified physical properties', *Applied Physics Letters,* 2006;**88**(10):102–103
12 Poulton A. 'Quantum tunnelling composite: touch and force sensing applications', *International Society for Prosthetics and Orthotics – Trent Prosthetic Symposium*, City Hospital Nottingham: United Kingdom, 2005, 5
13 Kyberd P., J. *Algorithmic Control of a Multifunction Hand Prosthesis*, PhD thesis, University of Southampton, 1990
14 Kyberd P. J. and Chappell P. H. 'Object-slip detection during manipulation using a derived force vector', *Mechatronics* 1992;**2**(1):1–13

Chapter 4
Control

A person wearing an artificial hand will want to control the movement of the fingers and thumb or generate grip force. They will need some device that could be an electronic, electromechanical or mechanical interface. The person may simply desire to open and close the hand. An electronic signal generated from some action by the person can be sent to the actuator(s) to cause the desired effect. A simple open-loop controller can be made to achieve such an action (Figure 4.1). For the position of the fingers to be controlled precisely requires a detailed mathematical model of all the parts of the system. The model parameters will need to be determined through measurements made on the components. Only then can precise control be achieved. However, most systems will have variable parameters such as friction and backlash in the finger mechanisms.

A much better idea is to use negative feedback shown in Figure 4.2. The advantages of using a feedback control system have been extensively researched. For the artificial hand, there are the advantages of improved performance in terms of making precise finger movements and automatic grips.

The person controlling an artificial hand can control posture and force generated in an open-loop way, but this would require continuous monitoring of the hand and have a cognitive burden. Adopting a hierarchical control structure frees the person of having to think all the time about state of the hand (Figure 4.3). The lower levels of control are automatic electronic systems, so that the person simply instructs the controller to instigate grip of an object and monitor any slipping that may occur. People who use an artificial hand would like to have some sensory feedback, i.e., be able to feel some property of an object such as surface texture. Here, sensors can estimate these physical properties and through the skin surface stimulate neurons to elicit a sense of feeling, i.e., haptic feedback.

4.1 Finger position

The analysis of the position control of a finger is presented in this section. The circuit diagram for a permanent magnet DC motor, with a mechanical load, is shown in Figure 4.4. The load on the motor is from the finger links, tip and bearings. There is also inertia and friction in the motor and its gearbox. The friction and inertia vary as a finger curls but can be combined and assumed to be constant.

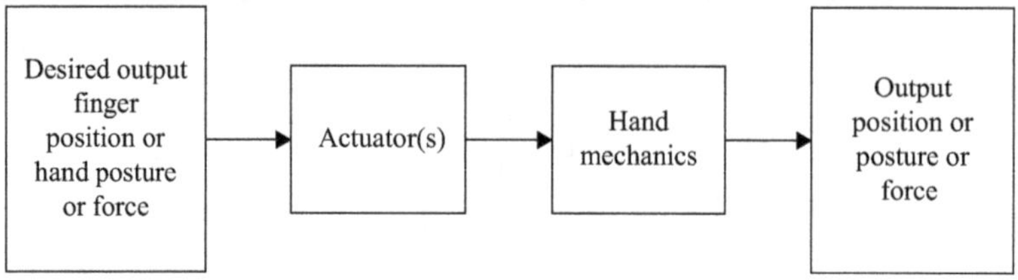

Figure 4.1 Open-loop control of a hand system with no feedback signals

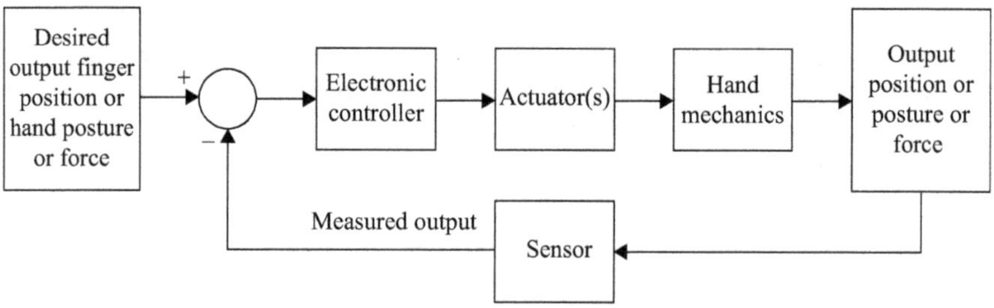

Figure 4.2 Closed-loop control of a hand system using negative feedback of measured output variable

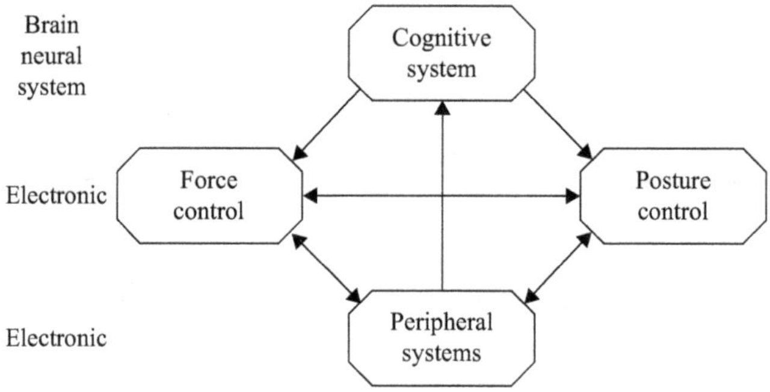

Figure 4.3 Hierarchical control

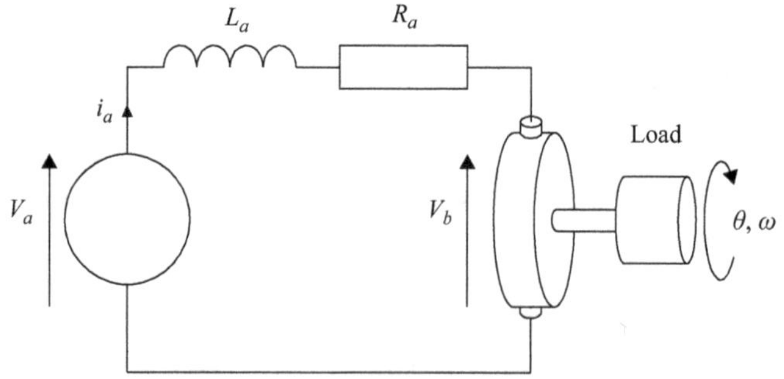

Figure 4.4 Permanent magnet DC motor

The electrical equation for the DC motor is

$$V_a = V_b + R_a i_a + L_a \frac{di_a}{dt} \tag{4.1}$$

where V_a is the applied armature voltage, V_b is the back emf voltage, R_a is the armature resistance, i_a is the armature current and L_a is the armature inductance.

The back emf voltage is dependent on the armature velocity

$$V_b = k_m \omega \tag{4.2}$$

where k_m is the back emf constant and ω the rotational velocity.

The load torque, T_l, is given by

$$T_l = J\frac{d^2\theta}{dt^2} + B\frac{d\theta}{dt} \tag{4.3}$$

where J is the moment of inertia, B is the friction constant and θ is the angle of the motor shaft and armature.

Taking Laplace transforms of the equations

$$V_a = V_b + R_a I_a + sL_a I_a \tag{4.4}$$

$$V_b = sk_m\theta \tag{4.5}$$

$$T_l = s^2 J\theta + sB\theta \tag{4.6}$$

Combining these equations to form the third-order transfer function, $G(s)$, relating the output position, θ, to the input voltage, V_a

$$\frac{\theta}{V_a} = \frac{k_m}{s\{(L_a s + R_a)(Js + B) + k_m^2\}} \tag{4.7}$$

The time constant for the motor (L_a/R) is usually small compared to the other system parameters, and hence the motor transfer function can be simplified to a first-order system

$$G(s) = \frac{k_m}{s\{R_a(Js + B) + k_m^2\}} \tag{4.8}$$

or

$$G(s) = \frac{k_0}{s(\tau_0 s + 1)} \tag{4.9}$$

where

$$k_0 = \frac{k_m}{(R_a B + k_m^2)} \tag{4.10}$$

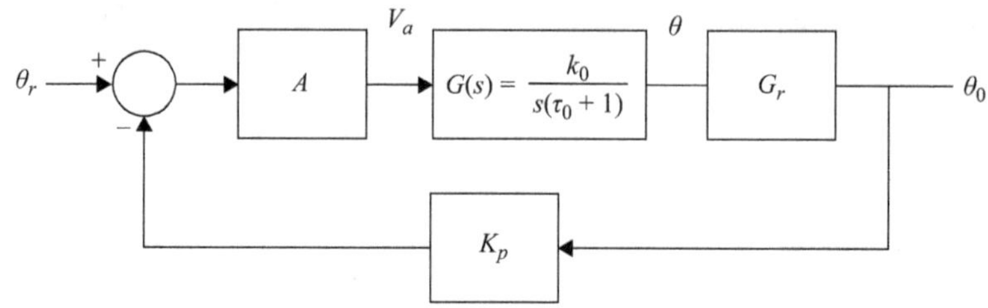

Figure 4.5 Closed-loop position control system for a finger

and

$$\tau_0 = \frac{R_a J}{(R_a J + k_m^2)} \tag{4.11}$$

A closed-loop system can be formed from the open-loop system given by (4.11) (Figure 4.5). The motor is supplied with power from an amplifier that has a gain, A, and a gearbox connects the output of the motor shaft (θ) to the finger shaft (θ_0). The demanded position of the finger, θ_r, is typically a processed signal from an electromyographic (EMG) amplifier. To form the closed loop, the signal from a position sensor with a gain, K_p is feedback to the summing point.

The open-loop transfer function for this system is

$$H(s)G(s) = \frac{Ak_0 G_r K_p}{\tau_0 s\left(s + \dfrac{1}{\tau_0}\right)} \tag{4.12}$$

where G_r is the gearbox ratio.

The parameters A and K_p can be adjusted to obtain the desired transient response. Figure 4.6 shows the root locus plot for the system where there are two poles. A critically damped response can be achieved if the gain is increased to the point where the two poles meet along the real axis at $-\frac{1}{2\tau_0}$. Alternatively the gain can be further increased, so that the response is under-damped resulting in a faster response with some overshoot.

The closed-loop system can be improved further by using a standard three-term controller that has proportional, integral and differential components (PID) (Figure 4.7).

The output of the PID controller is given by

$$\text{PID output} = K_p e + K_i \int e\,dt + K_d \frac{de}{dt} \tag{4.13}$$

here K_p, K_i and K_d are the gains of the three terms and the error, e is given by the difference between the input reference angle, θ_r, and the output shaft angle, θ_0

$$e = \theta_r - \theta_0 \tag{4.14}$$

The parameters can be determined by different methods to find a solution for the desired response to this search problem in the three-dimensional space of K_p, K_i and K_d.

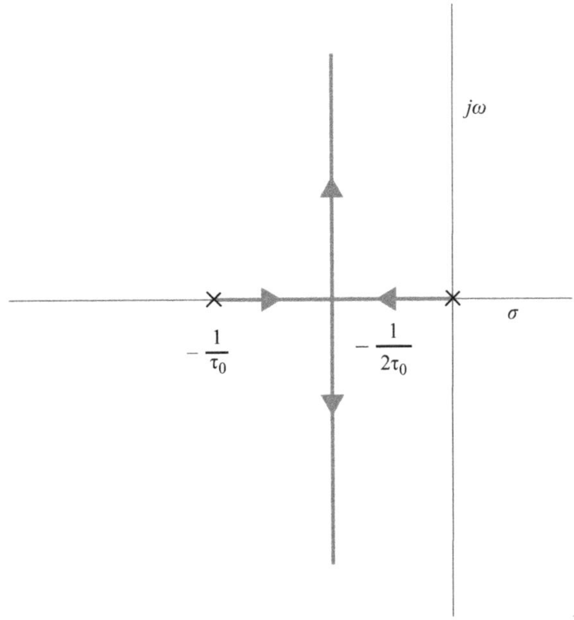

Figure 4.6 Root locus plot for the closed-loop system

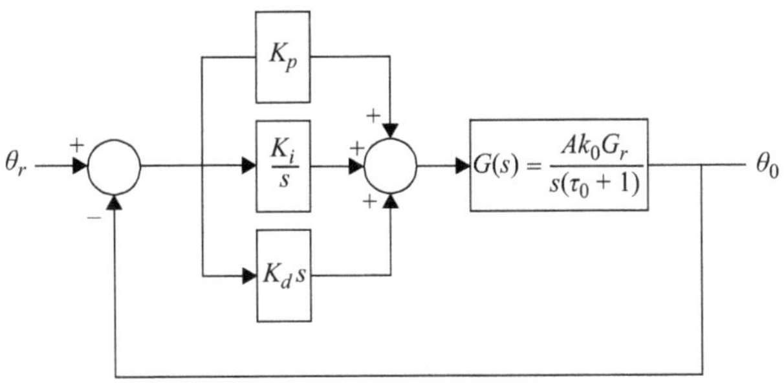

Figure 4.7 A position control system with a PID controller

It may not be necessary to have all three terms for a satisfactory performance. For a small or zero steady-state error the integral term is required with the differential term removed.

For a simple finger attached to the shaft, the position of a fingertip relative to a solid palm is also linearly related to the angle of the shaft. Where there is a nonlinear relationship between the shaft angle and the fingertip, the performance of a controller may vary depending on the shaft angle and fingertip position. However, this variation may be slight if the controller parameters are selected to minimise the effects of the nonlinearity. Alternatively an adaptive controller can be designed where parameters are updated from shaft position information.

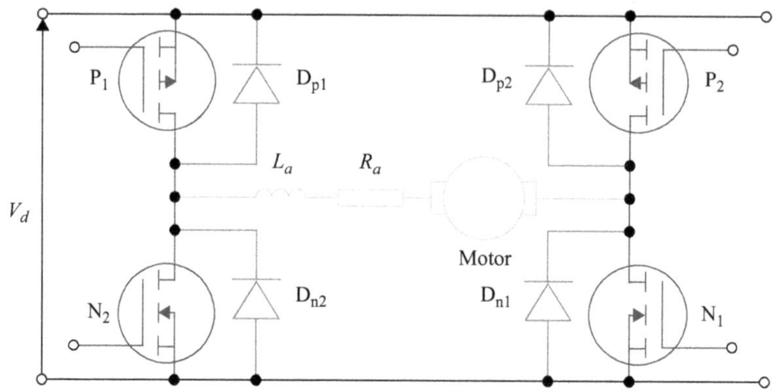

Figure 4.8 H-bridge for powering a DC motor

Power from a battery is typically supplied at 6 V, and an H-bridge is used to control a DC motor (Figure 4.8). This power electronic circuit has four transistors that are typically MOSFETs with two P-channel devices located at the top of the circuit and two N-channel ones at the bottom. In parallel with each transistor is a diode that is used to return current from the motor to the battery. There may be energy stored in the armature inductance or the motor can act as a generator converting mechanical energy into electrical energy. If there are no diodes, then the transistors may experience high voltages across their drain/source terminals which will lead to unreliable operation and ultimately the destruction of the devices. In its simplest operation, if the pair of transistors P_1 and N_1 is turned on, current flows from the battery through the motor and torque is generated in the motor shaft. Turning off this pair and turning on the pair, P_2 and N_2 causes the opposite polarity of battery voltage to be applied to the motor. Torque in the motor shaft and hence the direction of rotation and either flexing or extending a finger can be achieved. However, in operation, the circuit is more complex than this simple mode of forward-stop-reverse. It is necessary to wait until all the current has decayed away, and the motor is stationary before reversing the direction of torque/rotation. Otherwise, there is the possibility of shoot through where, e.g., P_1 and N_2 are on together causing the battery to be short circuited. Another possibility is where the motor is run at maximum velocity (no-load) and then the controller demands full rotation in the opposite direction. Under these circumstances, there is about twice the battery voltage across the motor and hence twice the expected stall current (approximately 2 V_d/R_a). This current may return to the supply through diodes. The transistors may have been specified to handle the stall current (the maximum expected), but the diodes may not be able to withstand twice this value. Also, typically the voltage across a diode is 0.7 V, which is larger than that when the MOSFET is saturated (typically 0.1 V). Consequently the power dissipated in the transistor may be almost an order of magnitude bigger than that dissipated in the diode resulting in the destruction of the power semiconductor. There are many more combinations of switching the transistors, which are not described here. For example, if the transistors P_1 and N_1 are turned on and current flows through the motor armature and then P_1 is turned off, current will circulate round through the motor, N_1 and the diode D_{n2}. The power dissipated in D_{n2} can be reduced by turning on N_2. Control of the mean voltage across the motor is achieved using pulse-width-modulation (PWM) where a rectangular voltage at a fixed frequency is applied. By varying the mark–space ratio the mean voltage can be controlled. However, applying a step input of voltage to a stationary DC motor causes the armature current, i_a, to rise and vary exponentially with time.

$$i_a = \frac{V_d}{R_a}\left(1 - \exp\left(\frac{-tR_a}{L_a}\right)\right) \tag{4.15}$$

If the switching frequency is high enough, then the ripple or rise (and fall) in current is small. However, the time constant (L_a/R_a) of small DC motors is such that the current will reach the stall value before the voltage is removed in a PWM cycle. Hence the current will be almost a square wave rather than a triangular wave. To overcome this problem, either the PWM frequency is increased or an inductor is added in series with the motor. Obviously, adding an inductor is not desirable as this extra component adds mass and increases the size of the power converter.

4.2 Object slip

To grip automatically requires information from the relative movement between an object and part of a hand such as a finger or thumb tip. The slip signal is processed, and a control algorithm put into action to arrest the slide.

Todd [1] proposed a control law that increases the grip force to stop an object sliding. The properties of the object surface or its mass are unknown, and therefore it is not possible to predict the grip force. A minimum force from the fingers (mg), just large enough to stop sliding, is required to balance the gravitational force from the mass of the object. The control law is

$$F = ky \tag{4.16}$$

where F is the grip force on the object, k is a constant and y is the total slip distance.

The distance can be found by measuring the relative velocity, v_r, between the fingers and object.

$$x = \int_0^{t_1} v_r \, dt \tag{4.17}$$

where t_1 is the time at which slipping ceases.

Ideally the signal from a slip sensor measures this velocity and is positive (the distance is always increasing). The distance is then easily calculated by a digital processor using a Cote's formula, e.g., Simpson's formula.

$$\int_{t_0}^{t_2} v_r \, dt \approx (t_2 - t_0)\left(\frac{1}{6}v_0 + \frac{4}{6}v_1 + \frac{1}{6}v_2\right) \tag{4.18}$$

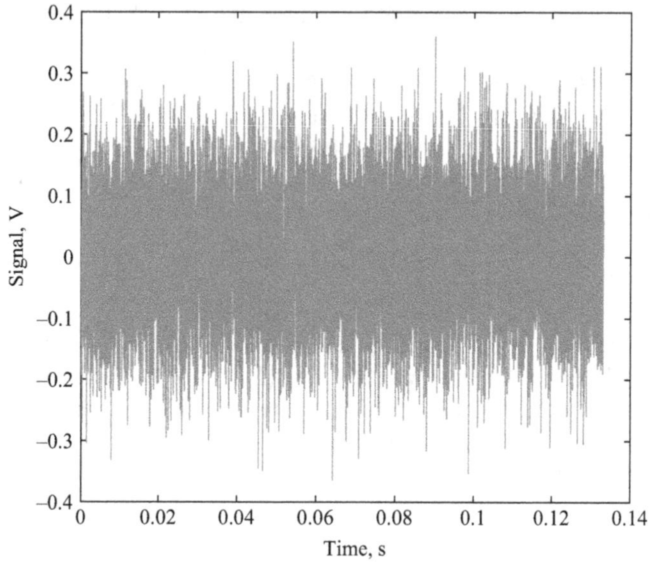

Figure 4.9 A random and normally distributed signal with zero mean and a standard deviation of 0.1

The control law can be approximated by

$$R = k\int_0^{t_1} v_s \, dt \tag{4.19}$$

where R is the reaction force on the object being gripped, k is a constant and v_s is the sensor slip signal.

A practical slip signal, from a sensor, is typically AC showing that there is movement of the object but with no DC component that indicates information about the direction of travel, i.e., movement in either the positive or the negative direction. A typical signal can be noisy as shown in Figure 4.9, which is a simulated random and normal distribution of a noise signal with zero mean and a standard deviation of 0.1. A simple method for implementing (4.19) first proposed by Todd requires rectification and thresholding of a signal (Figure 4.10) to form discrete values for counting. A '1' is recorded when the rectified signal traverses the set threshold (Figure 4.11). Figure 4.12 shows the accumulation of '1' s over time. The summed counts as a function of time are very linear as indicated by the high R-square value.

Alternatively the integration can be replaced by the summation over the time intervals, j, and sliding stops at the nth sample.

$$x_n = \sum_{j=0}^{n} d_{sj} \tag{4.20}$$

where x_n is the slip distance at the nth time interval and d_{sj}, the digital signal is either '1' or '0' at the jth count.

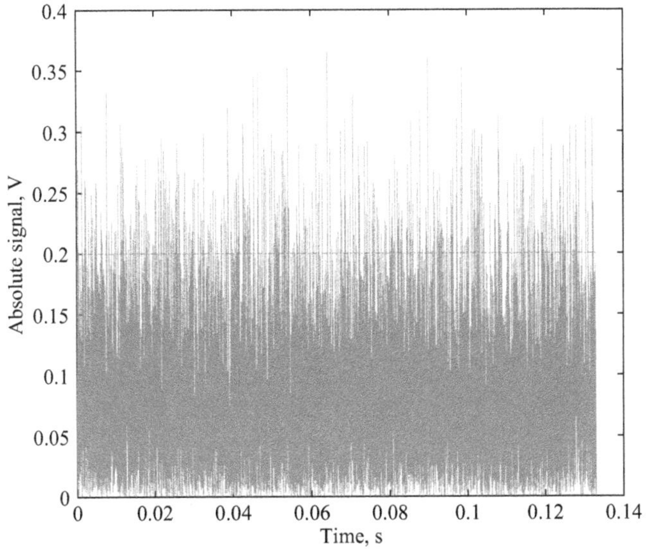

Figure 4.10 Rectified signal from Figure 4.9 with a threshold set at 0.2

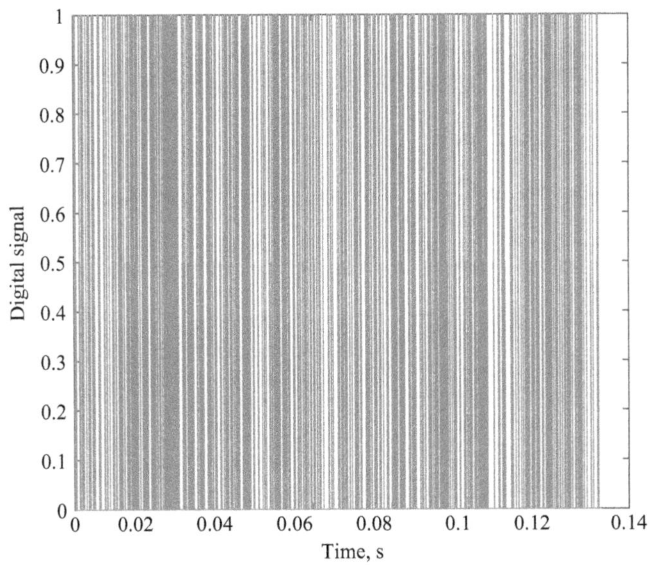

Figure 4.11 The digital signal for counting. A value of '1' occurs every time the rectified signal traverses the 0.2 threshold

The effect of varying the threshold can be seen in Figure 4.13, where there is a high correlation below about a threshold of 0.3. Therefore, the method is very tolerant to the setting of the threshold value. The intercept of the regression of the accumulated counts with time varies by a small amount (Figure 4.14), whereas the slope decreases as the threshold increases (Figure 4.15).

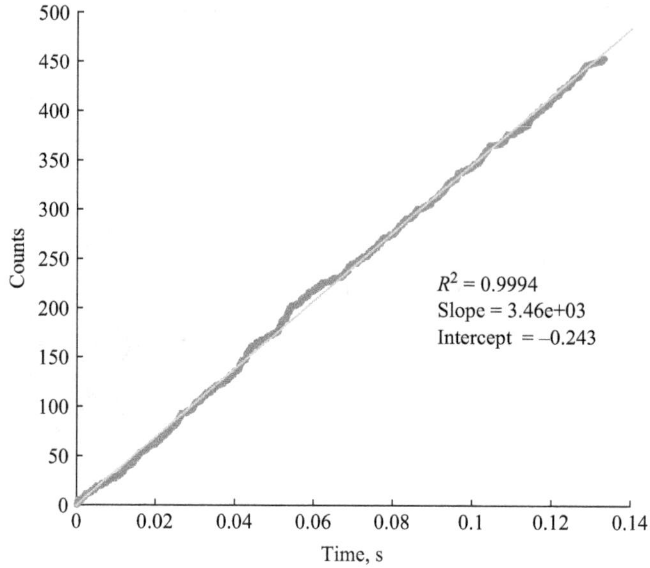

Figure 4.12 Accumulated counts showing a high linear relationship with time

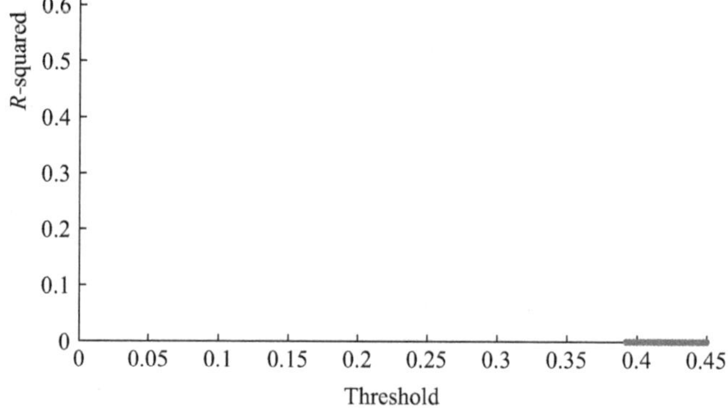

Figure 4.13 A plot showing the effect on R-squared of varying the threshold

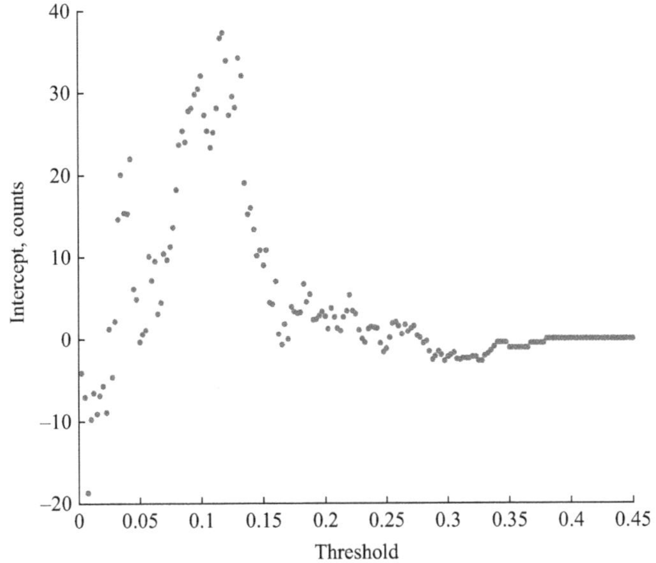

Figure 4.14 Intercept from a linear model when the threshold is varied

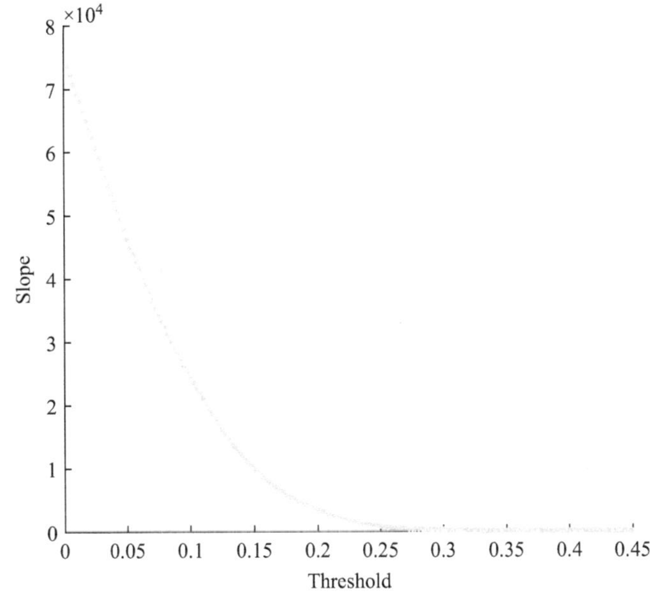

Figure 4.15 Slopes of a linear model as a function of threshold

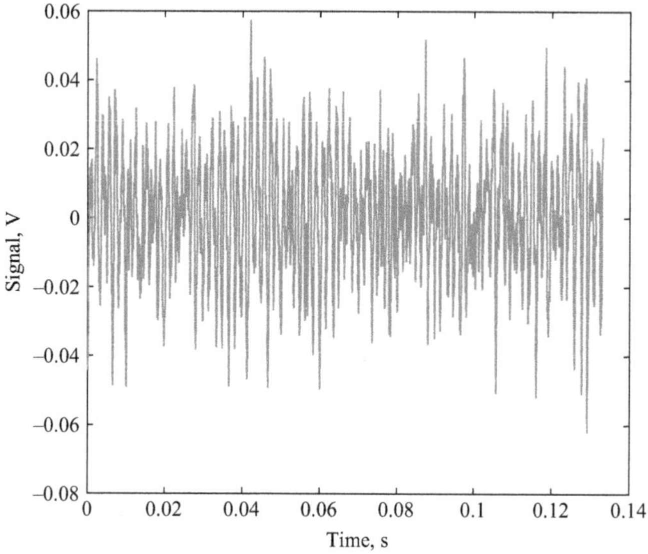

Figure 4.16 A slip signal from a repeating grating pattern

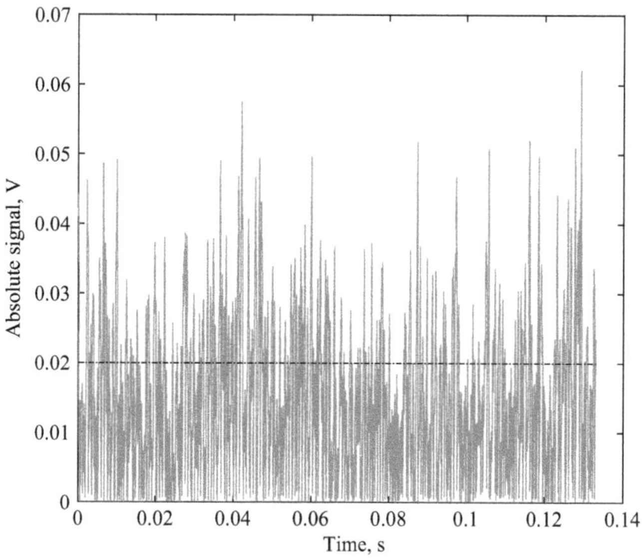

Figure 4.17 Rectified signal from Figure 4.16 with a threshold set at 0.02

The technique also functions in a similar manner for a real slip signal (Figures 4.16 to 4.22). This signal is from a piezoelectric fingertip sensor in contact with a surface that has a repeating pattern of 0.2 mm notches and 0.2 mm groves.

Should an absolute measure of distance be required, then any sensor would need to be calibrated and tested against different surface patterns on test objects,

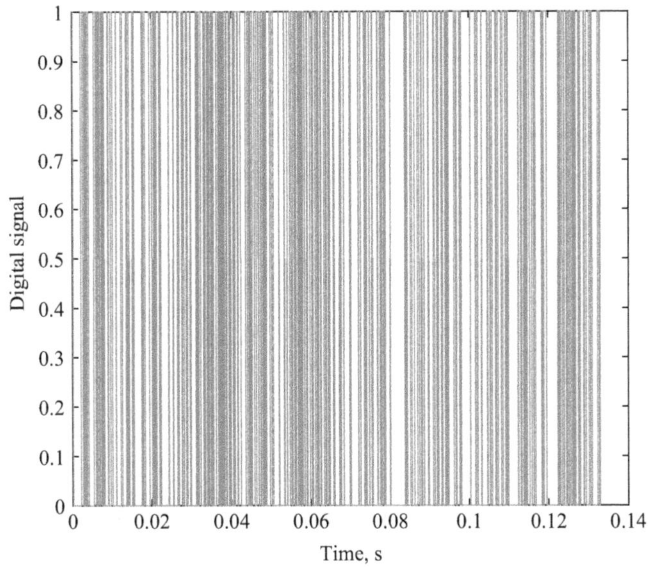

Figure 4.18 The digital signal for counting. A value of '1' occurs every time the rectified signal traverses the 0.2 threshold

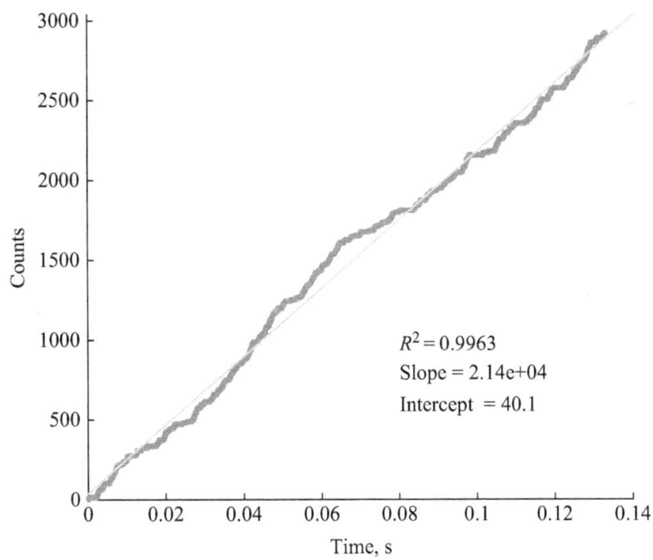

Figure 4.19 Accumulated counts showing a high linear relationship with time

since while the intercept can be ignored the slope of the relationship does vary with threshold.

Todd found that when sliding ceased, the force was larger than that needed to achieve weight balance. He proposed a modified law to improve the performance of the controller.

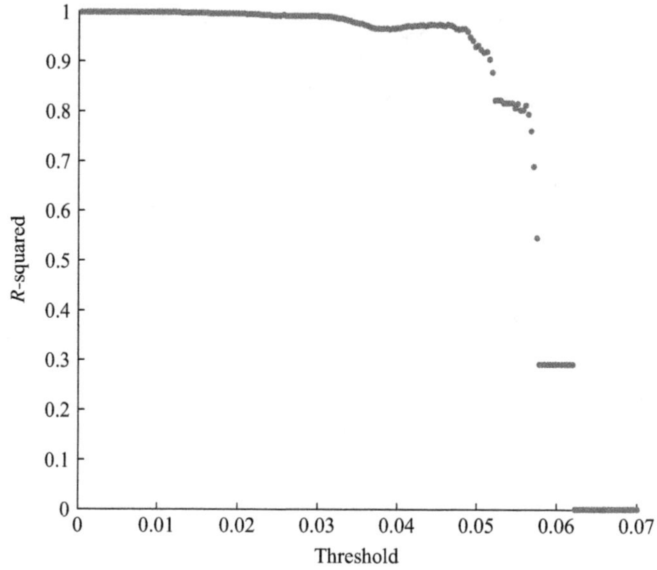

Figure 4.20 A plot showing the effect on R-squared of varying the threshold

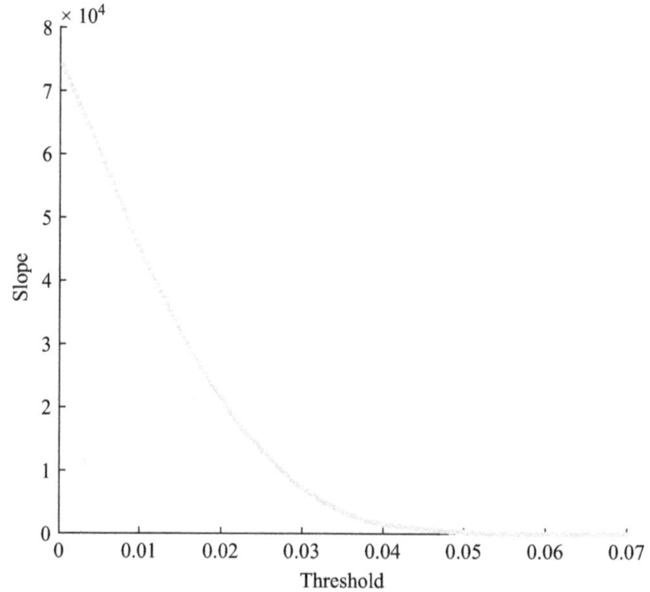

Figure 4.21 Slopes of a linear model as a function of threshold

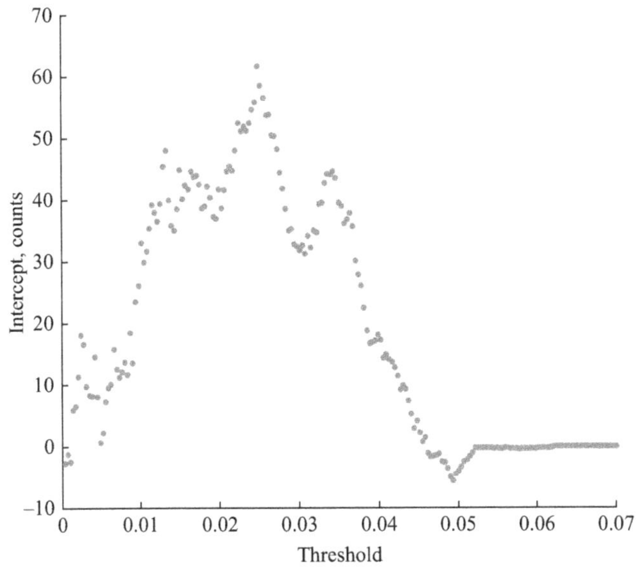

Figure 4.22 Intercept from a linear model when the threshold is varied

4.3 Reference inputs

In the traditional control engineering sense, any voltage input can be used as a reference input signal or demand signal to the positioning of a finger (Figure 4.2). For testing purposes, this input could be simply the output from a voltage divider circuit using a DC supply connected to a potentiometer adjusted manually by turning the wiper shaft. However, the prosthetic user needs to create signals from his or her body. Typically, these signals are EMG from surface electrodes placed on the skin above a residual muscle. Voluntary contraction of a skeletal muscle produces small voltages (approximately 1–10 μV) on the skin surface that can be amplified and conditioned.

A muscle contraction at its smallest level produces a twitch in muscle force. This small force is from a single motor unit. On producing another twitch, another motor unit contracts; the technical term for this is recruitment of motor units. To maintain a low constant force, motor units are recruited randomly. The force generation is not continuous but composed of a summation of twitches. It is the three-dimensional electrical activity of these motor units that appears as a potential difference between two electrodes attached to the skin surface. A diagrammatic representation of this process is shown in Figure 4.23. A demand for a muscle contraction begins with a signal from the brain being sent down the spinal cord. The electrical activity of the motor units travel through the tissues of the body, and it is the summation of this volume electrical activity that is detected at the skin surface. An EMG signal is intriguing as it appears to have some information about a muscle contraction. However, an analysis using approximate entropy shows that

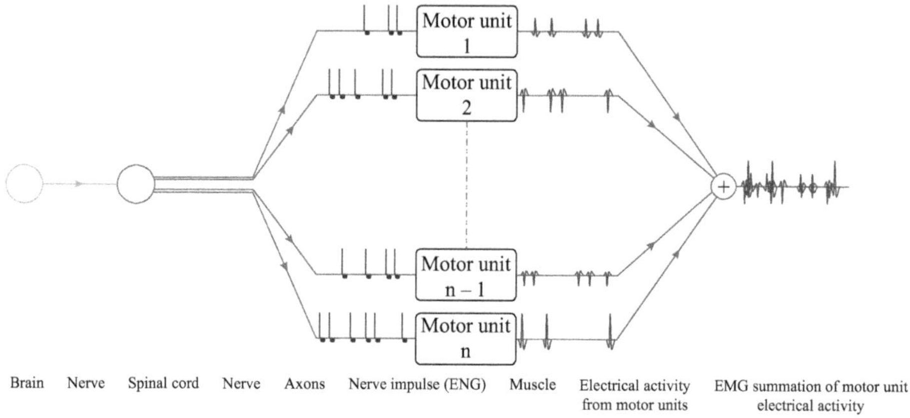

Figure 4.23 Diagrammatic block diagram of the formation of an EMG signal from the three-dimensional electrical activity of individual motor units

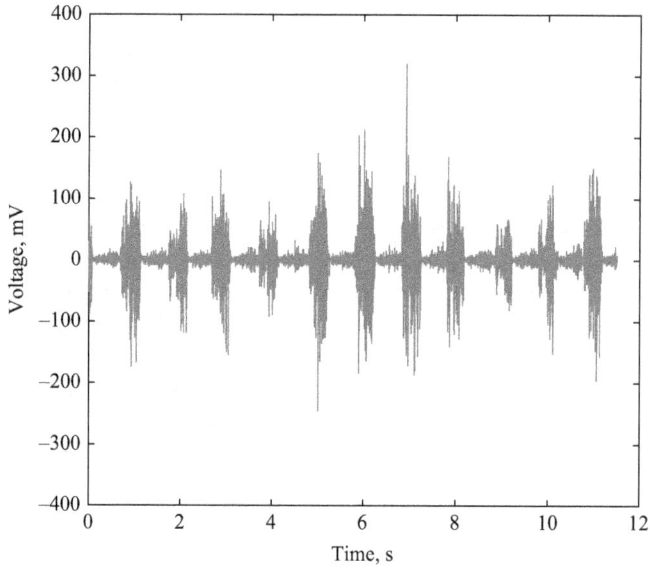

Figure 4.24 EMG signal showing eleven bursts of muscle activity

an EMG signal contains no signal information. When an isometric contraction is steady, then the average of the absolute EMG signal is approximately linearly related to the developed muscle force. An increase or decrease in EMG has information and has been used to train an artificial neural network for the control of artificial hands and the upper limb. The dynamic nature of an EMG signal can be used to track muscle force if an adaptive filter is used.

A sample of an EMG signal is shown in Figure 4.24 that is in bursts of contraction of a muscle in the forearm. The corresponding signal spectrum for an

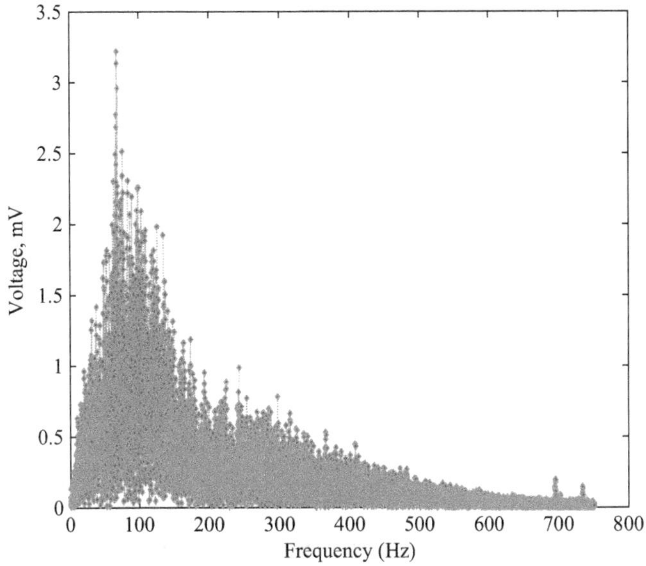

Figure 4.25 An analysis of the frequency components of the signal shown in Figure 4.24

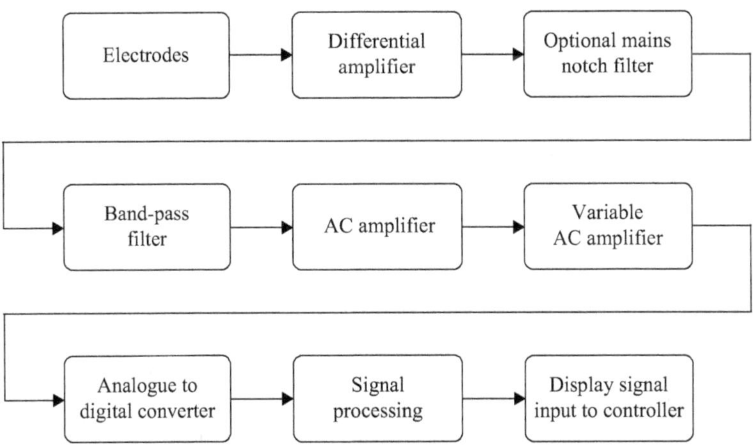

Figure 4.26 Block diagram of an EMG system

analysis of this signal using an FFT is shown in Figure 4.25. It can be seen in this plot that most of the signal has frequencies below 700 Hz and that the majority of the components are centred on about 60 Hz. Any notch filter, to remove mains interference at 60 or 50 Hz depending on the country, needs to have a high specification since its use will remove some of the EMG signal and cause some phase distortion.

A block diagram of the components to detect EMG signals is shown in Figure 4.26. The electrodes can be of various shapes but are typically of a regular

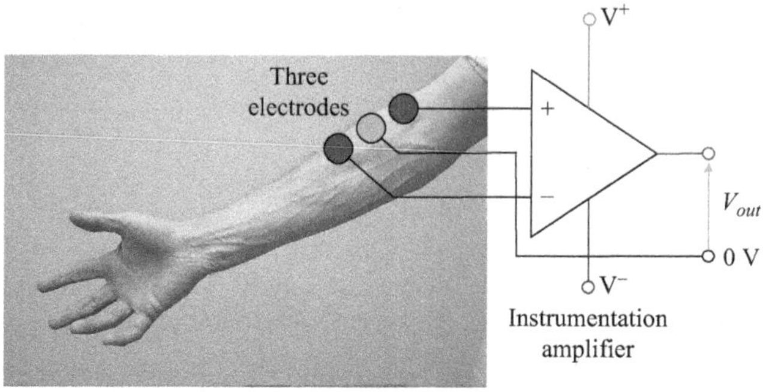

Figure 4.27 Attachment of three electrodes to a forearm and then to an instrumentation amplifier

shape or for circular types about 10 mm in diameter. They can be constructed from a metal such as stainless steel or brass and can be gold or silver plated. Also commercial electrodes that are flexible and made with a conductive gel (silver–silver chloride) can be used to observe an EMG signal. A differential amplifier with a high input impedance and common mode rejection ratio (CMRR of 120 dB) detects the tiny voltages on the skin surface (Figure 4.27). A typical instrumentation amplifier can be used with a small gain (about two). The CMRR may vary with gain and a small gain may maximise the CMRR, but too much gain may result in an unwanted and large mains interference signal. Three electrodes are used: two for the potential difference and one as a reference electrode, i.e., typically centrally located between the two signal electrodes. Depending on the electrical environment, a notch filter set at mains supply frequency (60 or 50 Hz) can be used to remove interference. Alternatively or as well the reference electrode can be driven in a feedback loop that is often found in a 'right-leg-driven' arrangement for the measurement of the electrocardiogram or ECG and improves the CMRR. The signal is then band limited from a few hertz to a kilohertz or more but as there is little signal in the EMG at the higher frequencies this may not be necessary unless there is high frequency noise present. Amplification of the signal further can be achieved with a simple AC amplifier (Figure 4.28). The gain is set by R_2/R_1 and the low frequency cut-off of the first order filter by $1/(2\pi R_1 C)$. In practise a gain of about ten is the highest achievable. The reason for this limit is that there is a design trade-off between selecting the values of the resistors and capacitor. High values of resistors maintain low-power consumption, but in general the larger the capacitance the larger is the physical size of the capacitor as it needs to be a bipolar variety. The low-frequency cut-off is reduced by increasing either R_1 or C. In order to have a low-frequency cut-off of around 10 Hz there is a limit in the size of the bipolar capacitors to about 1 μF. A second stage of amplification can be added to obtain a gain of 100.

The EMG signal can be processed in several ways. A simple method is to rectify and smooth the signal.

$$y(i) = |s(i)| \tag{4.21}$$

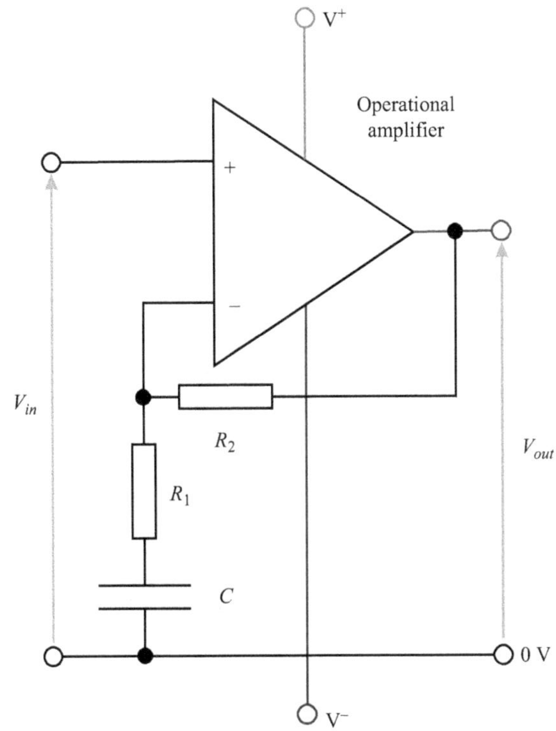

Figure 4.28 Non-inverting AC amplifier

where $s(i)$ is the EMG signal at time intervals i and $y(i)$ is the absolute signal.

The absolute signal can be smoothed with a moving average or weighted moving average.

$$\overline{y(t)} = \frac{\sum_{1}^{n} a_i y(i)}{n} \tag{4.22}$$

where a_i being the weights of the averaging process that can all be equal to 1 for a standard definition of the mean or typically of decreasing values from 1. Figure 4.29 shows the absolute values of the EMG signal shown in Figure 4.24. With equal weights, this signal can be smoothed with an averaging filter (Figure 4.30) and compared to a threshold; the digital signal when the absolute EMG signal is above the threshold is shown in Figure 4.30. If the averaging is calculated over too short a window, then there is uncertainty in the digital signal and feathering occurs (Figure 4.30). The feathering can be removed by choosing a longer averaging time as shown in Figure 4.31.

Perhaps a better method to extract a digital representation of the EMG signal activity is to use a leaky integrator where the processing switches depending on whether the signal is rising or falling. Applying a positive voltage to the input of the circuit, shown in Figure 4.32, causes current to flow into the capacitor and the

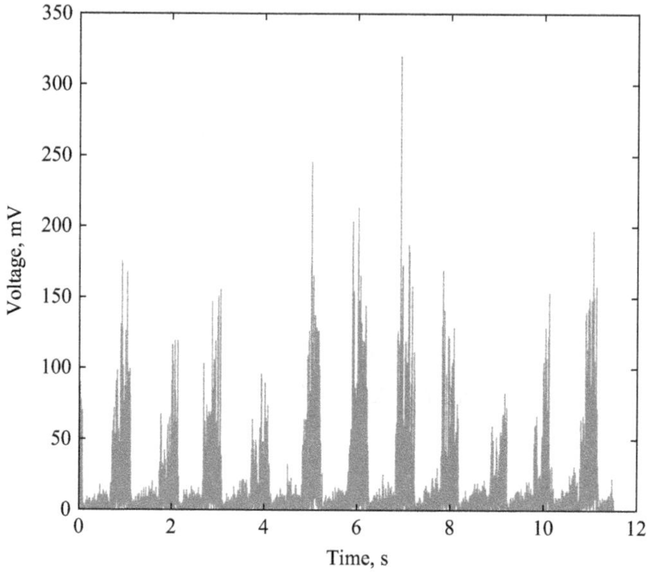

Figure 4.29 Absolute values of the EMG signal

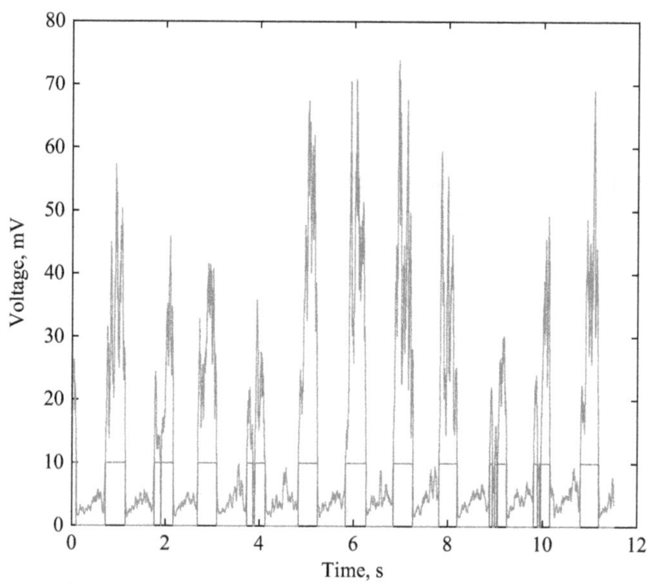

Figure 4.30 Smoothed signal with a window of length 33.3 ms and a digital signal produced by comparing it with a threshold of 10 mV. When the smoothed signal is above 10 mV a '1' is produced (shown in the figure as 10 mV). There is feathering of the digital signal around 2, 4, 9 and 10 s

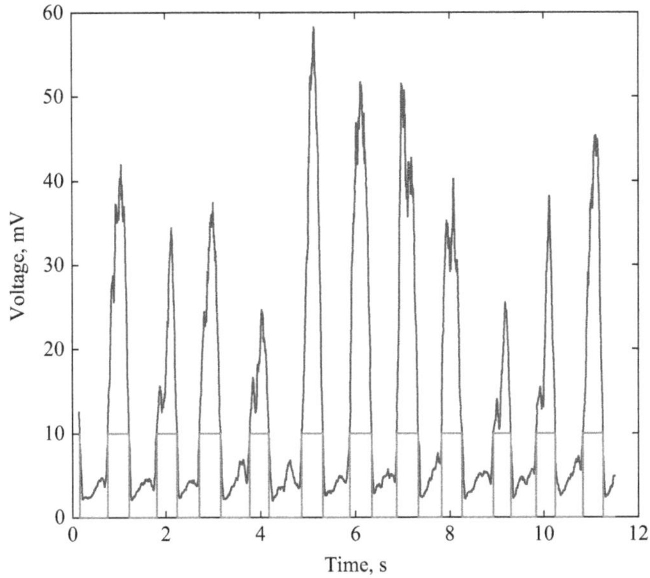

Figure 4.31 Smoothed signal with a window of length 133 ms and digital signal with a threshold of 10 mV

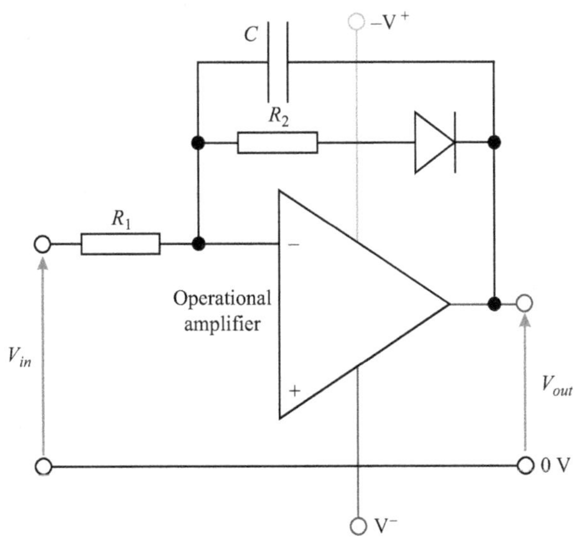

Figure 4.32 A circuit for a leaky integrator

output voltage will go negative. The diode is reverse biased and so the integration of the input signal is

$$V_o = \frac{1}{CR_1} \int V_i \, dt \tag{4.23}$$

A zero voltage applied to the input causes the diode to become forward biased and the voltage across the capacitor, and hence the output voltage to decay exponentially with time.

$$V_o = V_z \exp\left(\frac{-t}{CR_2}\right) \tag{4.24}$$

A slight variation on this integration is if the signal is rising, then integration occurs, whereas if it is falling then the output is a simple decay. This algorithm can be implemented digitally or using an analogue circuit as shown in Figure 4.32.

$$y = \int s \, dt \qquad \text{for} \qquad \frac{ds}{dt} > 0 \tag{4.25}$$

and

$$y = S_o \exp\left(\frac{-t}{\tau}\right) \qquad \text{for} \qquad \frac{ds}{dt} \leq 0 \tag{4.26}$$

where S_o is the initial value of s on switching from (4.25). In the processing, if the previous sample of the EMG signal, s, is greater than the current sample then the signal is integrated, otherwise it decays as a first-order system with a time constant, τ. Under the latter process the initial value is the last value of the integration and is therefore independent of the EMG signal.

Once an EMG has been smoothed, it can be compared to a threshold and a digital train of pulses generated (Figure 4.33). Figure 4.34 shows the scaled EMG and digital output from the processed data. This sequence of digital pulses can then be used in a state-driven algorithm to move the hand into different grip postures or control states.

Another method is to process the time sequence of EMG data using a moving measure of the Shannon entropy as defined by

$$E = -\sum_{i}^{n} {p_i}^2 \log {p_i}^2 \tag{4.27}$$

where p_i is the probability of the ith value occurring in the data. By calculating the entropy over the first $(1, \ldots, n)$ data values and then moving along by one value and recalculating over the next $(2, \ldots, n+1)$ values and so on, a moving entropy output can be determined. Figure 4.35 shows the result of this process for the EMG signal in Figure 4.24. Figure 4.36 shows the scaled EMG signal to compare it to the processed digital signal. The EMG data do not have to be rectified. Using more samples in the window results in a smoother entropy output, and hence the likelihood of spurious

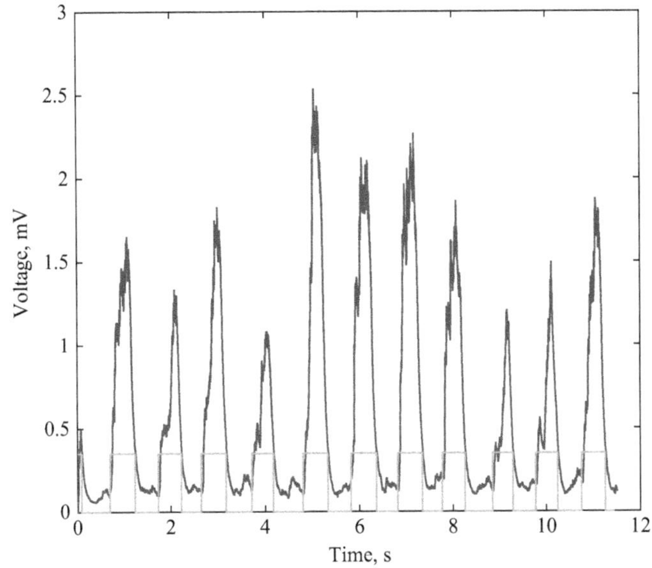

Figure 4.33 Processing of the EMG signal using the leaky integrator. The comparator threshold is 0.35 mV producing a train of digital pulses

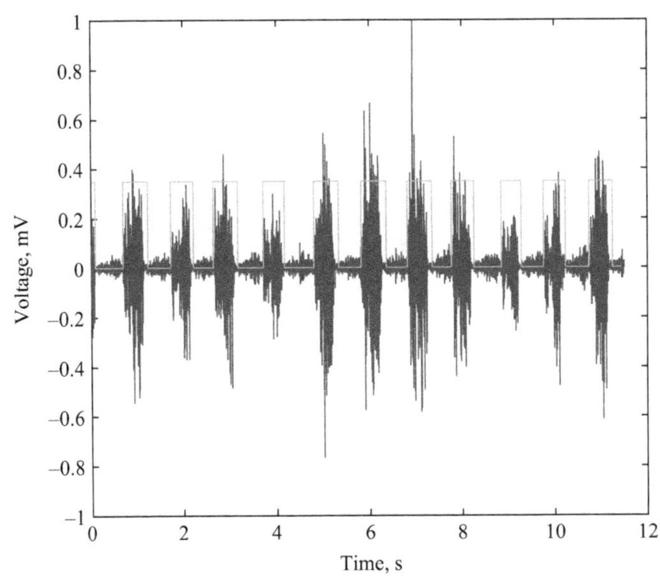

Figure 4.34 EMG signal (scaled to its maximum value) and output from the processed signal using a leaky integrator algorithm

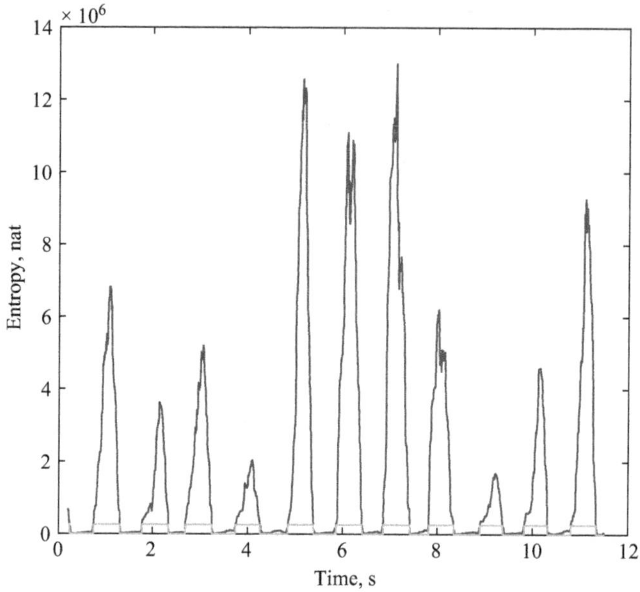

Figure 4.35 *Moving entropy processed EMG signal and digital output. Note that for convenience the entropy is negative but has been presented in this figure as positive values. The window is 300 samples that is 200 ms. The entropy threshold is* 2.5×10^5

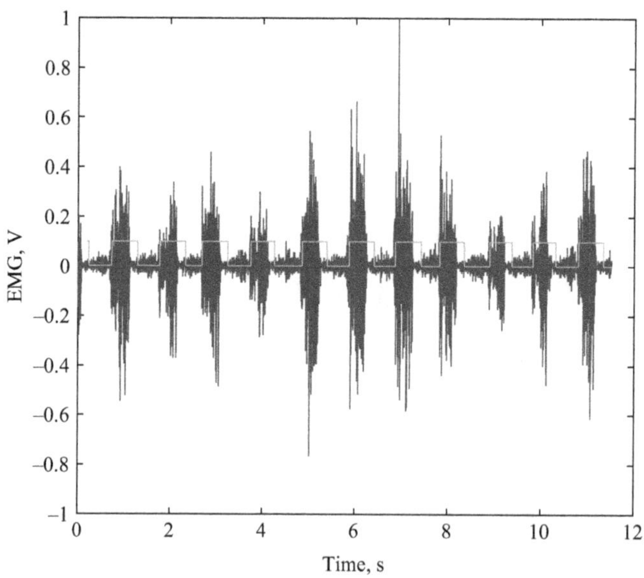

Figure 4.36 *EMG signal (scaled to its maximum value) and output from the processed signal using moving entropy*

transitions from zero to one and one to zero is reduced in the digital output with a selected threshold. However, there is a compromise as there is a delay in the processed output that is the time taken to calculate the entropy of the set window size. Also by taking the natural logarithm of the entropy calculated from (4.27), a possibly more robust digital output is achieved (Figures 4.37 and 4.38).

A person operating an artificial hand can use the digital sequence from a processed EMG signal to switch from one state to another such as the Southampton Adaptive Manipulation Scheme, SAMS, proposed by Kyberd. Figure 4.39 shows a sequence of such states starting in the centre where the hand is in a flat posture, i.e., all the fingers are fully extended away from the palm and the thumb is rotated and flexed to the lateral side of the first finger. By a digital sequence of two EMG signals from, e.g., flexor and extensor muscles, the hand fingers and thumb can be coordinated into several different hand postures. On receiving power from the battery, the controller moves the hand into the flat hand posture. By applying a digital flexion signal followed by a digital extension signal and a further flexion signal, the controller moves the hand into a full tips posture, precision, P_0. Here the fingers flex and extend together with the thumb opposing the midline between the first and second fingers. The hand can also be configured into two other precision postures, P_1 and P_2. In the first of these, the middle, third and little fingers are flexed into the palm and the first finger and thumb oppose each other at their tips. The second posture is the

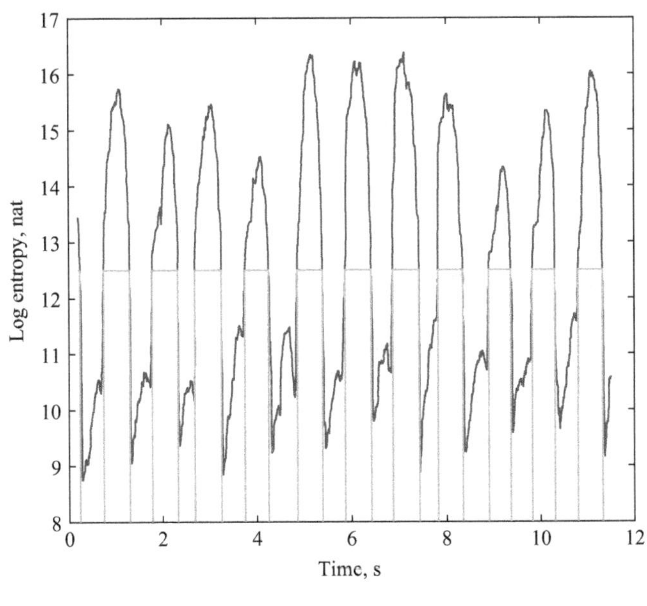

Figure 4.37 Natural logarithm of the moving entropy processed EMG signal and digital output. Note that for convenience the entropy is negative but has been presented in this figure as positive values. The window is 300 samples that is 200 ms. The entropy threshold is 12.5

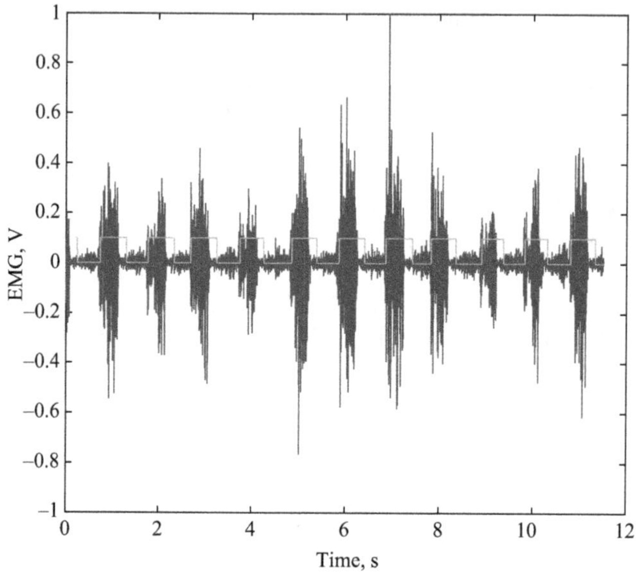

Figure 4.38 EMG signal (scaled to its maximum value) and output from the processed signal using log moving entropy

same as the first but the middle, third and little fingers are fully extended away from the palm. In P_1 and P_2, two-point grips are formed. These grips can be selected by the user generating a large flexion signal and then relaxing into one of two lower signals where the controller switches the hand into either P_1 or P_2. After selecting a desired posture the extensor signal is used to position the fingers and thumb. Increasing the extensor signal opens the hand by extending the fingers and thumb. They can then close an object by relaxing the extensor muscle. Once contact is made with the object the touch sensors stop the motors (touch state in Figure 4.39). A flexion digital signal will then place the controller in the hold state where the grip on the object is under automatic control using slip sensors mounted on the fingers and thumb. The object can be squeezed by producing a further flexion signal and then released by the generation of an extension signal. In this way, using series of digital signals such as those shown in Figure 4.37, a person can select different hand postures and move around the sequences shown in Figure 4.39. Different sequences to the ones described above can be implemented by selecting combinations of the two EMG signals. It is important to avoid any mechanical clash between the fingers and thumb, so the controller has to maintain an awareness of the spatial restrictions of the fingers and thumb created from the mechanical design. For example a hand could be placed in a small fist grip where the fingers are fully flexed and the thumb in then flexed over the top of them. If a flat hand is then requested, the controller must first extend the thumb out of the way of the fingers before they are flexed. Ambroise Paré had similar limitations to grip postures that can be formed with the handmade in the sixteenth century (see Chapter 1).

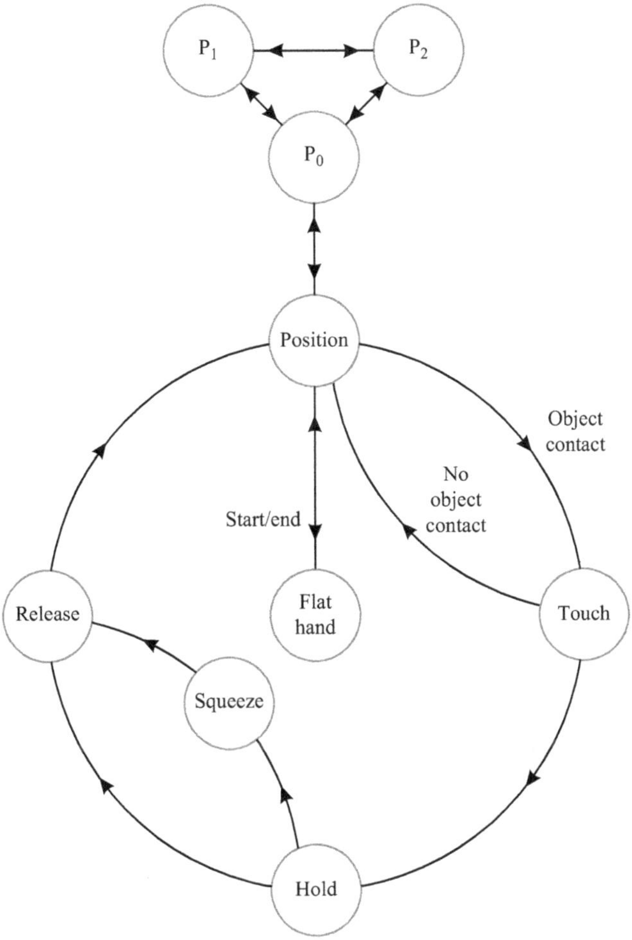

Figure 4.39 States in the Southampton Adaptive Manipulation Scheme, SAMS

4.4 Artificial prehension

In simple terms, the diagram in Figure 4.40 shows an object that is clamped between a fingertip and thumb. By controlling the input, u, the reaction at the contact surfaces, R, can be varied and the object held with a gentle grip or maximum grip force. The object can be allowed to slip downwards by controlling the grip force.

If the object is sliding, then its movement can be stopped by applying a suitable control input, u. How this input is adjusted depends on the applied control law.

There is the vertical force on the object, mg, from the Earth's gravitational field and any external force, P. The clamp applies a vertical force on the object depending on the reaction, R and the coefficient of friction, μ, between the object and clamp surfaces.

$$F = \mu R \tag{4.28}$$

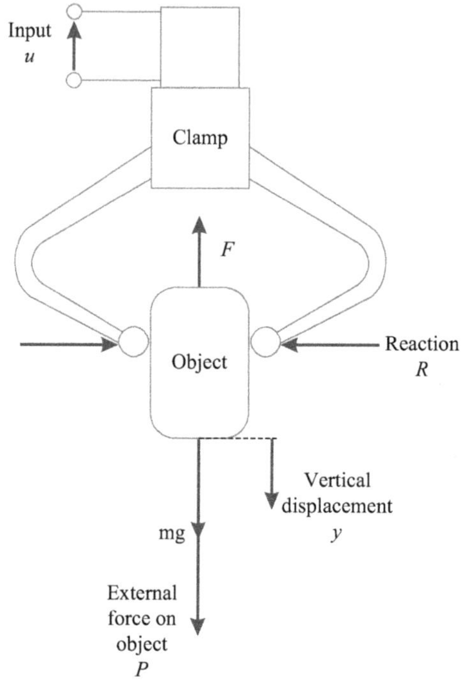

Figure 4.40 Object held in a clamp

The object motion is governed by

$$m\frac{d^2y}{dt^2} = mg - F + P \tag{4.29}$$

The object can be arrested in a specified distance, $(y_1 - y_0)$ or time, $(t_1 - t_0)$, by applying the control law

$$R = ky = k\int_{t_0}^{t_1}\frac{dy}{dt}dt \tag{4.30}$$

where k is a constant and the initial velocity is $\frac{dy}{dt}(t_0)$ and the final velocity $\frac{dy}{dt}(t_1)$ are zero.

If the external force, P, is zero, then the solution of the combining the dynamics (4.25) with the control law (4.26) is

$$\frac{d^2y}{dt^2} = g - \frac{F}{m} \tag{4.31}$$

$$\frac{d^2y}{dt^2} = g - \frac{\mu ky}{m} \tag{4.32}$$

Taking Laplace transforms

$$s^2Y = \frac{g}{s} - \frac{\mu kY}{m} \tag{4.33}$$

$$Y = \frac{g}{s\left(s^2 + \frac{\mu k}{m}\right)} \tag{4.34}$$

or

$$y = \frac{mg}{\mu k}\left(1 - \cos\sqrt{\frac{\mu k}{m}}t\right) \tag{4.35}$$

Differentiating this equation, the velocity is

$$\frac{dy}{dt} = g\sqrt{\frac{m}{\mu k}}\sin\sqrt{\frac{\mu k}{m}}t \tag{4.36}$$

The force on the object, F is

$$F = mg\left(1 - \cos\sqrt{\frac{\mu k}{m}}t\right) \tag{4.37}$$

The characteristics of the slip are illustrated in Figures 4.41 to 4.46 for a mass, m, of 0.1 kg, a coefficient of friction, μ, between the object and gripping surface of

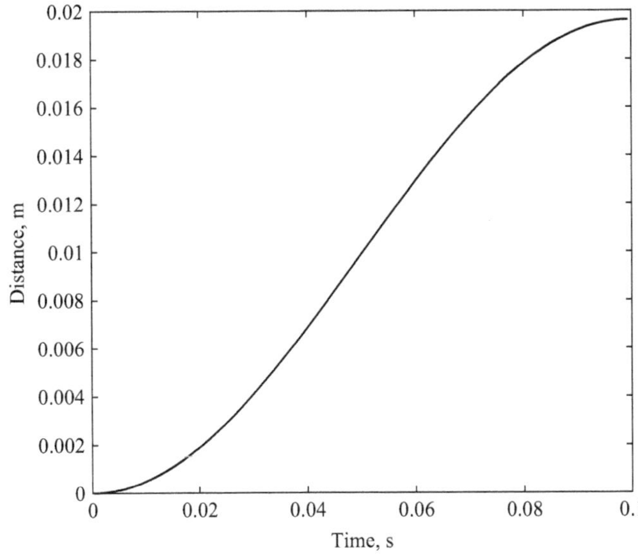

Figure 4.41 Distance travelled by object

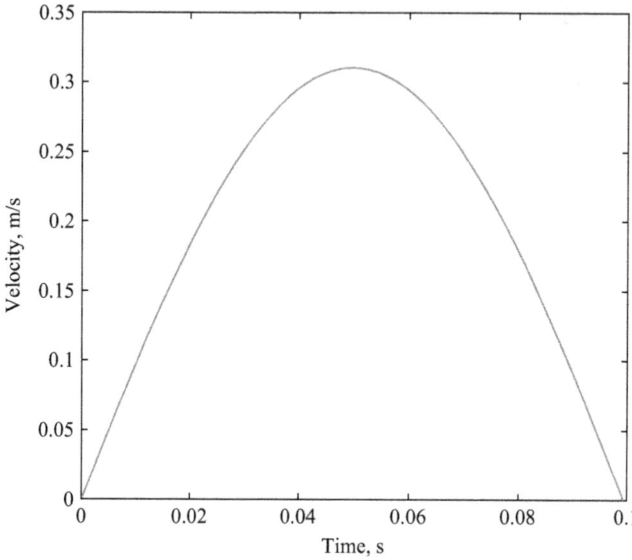

Figure 4.42 Velocity of object

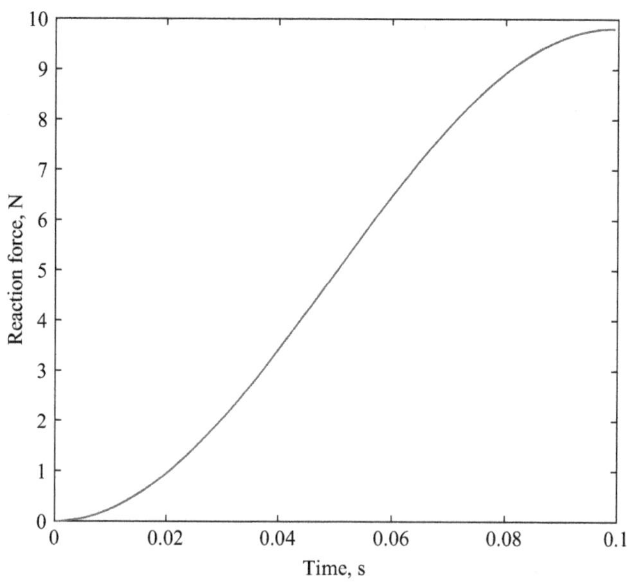

Figure 4.43 Reaction force

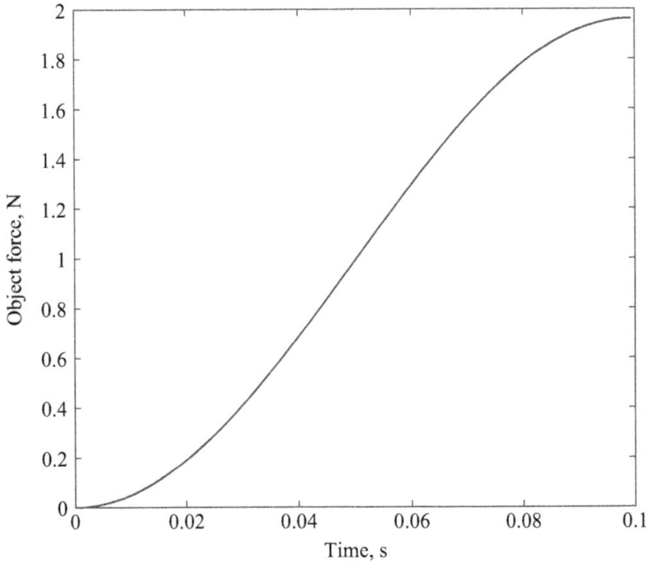

Figure 4.44 Object force

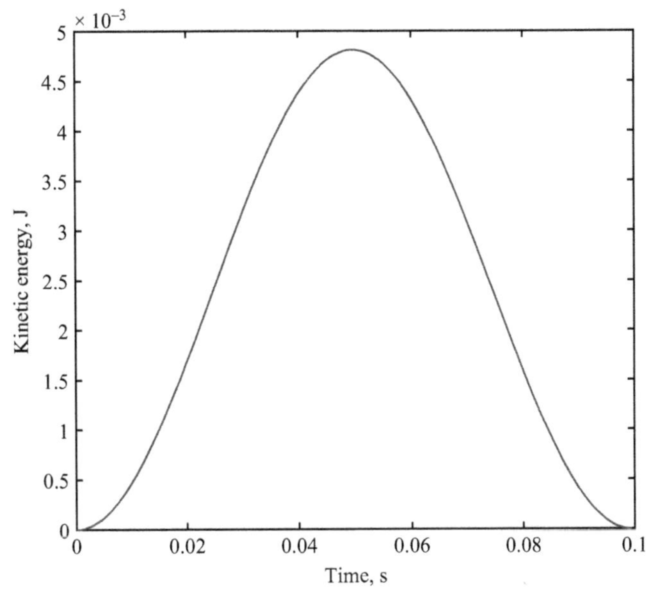

Figure 4.45 Kinetic energy

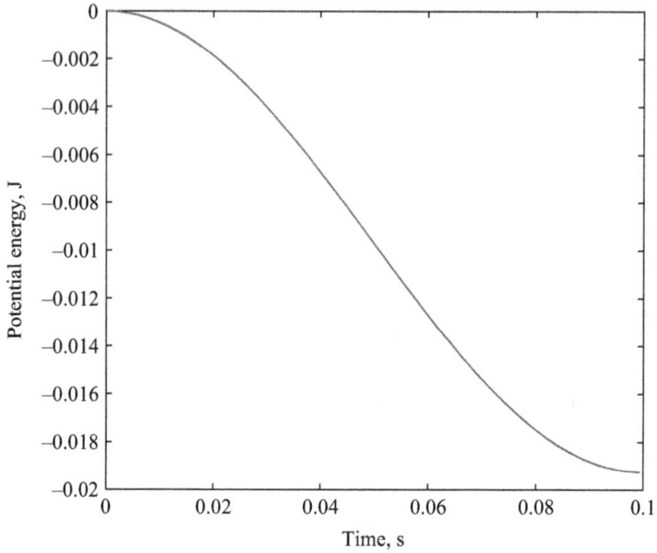

Figure 4.46 Potential energy

0.2 and a constant, k, for the control law of 500. The 100 g object has slipped a distance of about 20 mm and has been arrested with a force of about 2 N.

When the velocity zero at time, t_1, then

$$0 = g\sqrt{\frac{m}{\mu k}}\sin\sqrt{\frac{\mu k}{m}}t \tag{4.38}$$

The sine term is zero

$$\sqrt{\frac{\mu k}{m}}t_1 = \pi \tag{4.39}$$

or

$$t_1 = \pi\sqrt{\frac{m}{\mu k}} \tag{4.40}$$

At this time the distance moved is

$$y(t_1) = 2g\sqrt{\frac{m}{\mu k}} \tag{4.41}$$

And the force on the object is

$$F(t_1) = 2\,mg \tag{4.42}$$

Hence the object is always over gripped by a factor of two. To prevent the object from moving, once slipping has ceased, only requires a vertical force of mg to overcome that due to the gravitational field.

Changing the value of the control law constant, k, alters the time taken to arrest the object and also the distance travelled. Increasing k nonlinearly decreases the time taken and the slip distance. A similar relationship holds for the coefficient of friction, μ.

The reaction force, R is

$$R = ky = \frac{mg}{\mu}\left(1 - \cos\sqrt{\frac{\mu k}{m}}t\right) \tag{4.43}$$

The kinetic energy, e_k

$$e_k = \frac{1}{2}m\left(\frac{dy}{dt}\right)^2 \tag{4.44}$$

$$e_k = \frac{m^2g^2}{2\,\mu k}\sin^2\sqrt{\frac{\mu k}{m}}t \tag{4.45}$$

where the peak in energy occurs at $t_1/2$

$$e_k\left(\frac{t_1}{2}\right) = \frac{m^2g^2}{2\,\mu k} \tag{4.46}$$

The potential energy, e_p is

$$e_p = -mgy \tag{4.47}$$

When the object is arrested, at time t_1

$$e_p\left(\frac{t_1}{2}\right) = -\frac{2m^2g^2}{\mu k} \tag{4.48}$$

At time, t_1, the object is stationary when the velocity is zero and therefore

$$0 = g\cos\sqrt{\frac{\mu k}{m}}t_1 \tag{4.49}$$

$$\sqrt{\frac{\mu k}{m}}t_1 = \frac{\pi}{2} \tag{4.50}$$

or

$$t_1 = \frac{\pi}{2}\sqrt{\frac{m}{\mu k}} \tag{4.51}$$

Other control laws for proximity detection, holding, weight balance, manoeuvring and contouring of held objects have been investigated [1, 2].

4.5 Summary

Control of an artificial hand should be considered in closed-loop form to achieve good performance of positioning for the fingers and thumb. A demanded input position of a finger can be formed by processing the very small electrical signals from muscles. Electrodes attached to the skin surface pick up these signals that are then amplified and processed. Several mathematical and algorithmic techniques such as entropy and thresholding can be used successfully to control finger movement. Implementing a state-driven and hierarchal control law in a microcontroller and embedding it in the socket fitting the user's stump allows for the selection of a variety of different grip postures.

References

1 Todd R. W. *Adaptive Control of a Hand Prosthesis*, PhD thesis, University of Southampton, 1971

2 Baits J. C., Todd R. W., and Nightingale J. M. 'The feasibility of an adaptive control scheme for artificial prehension', *The Institution of Mechanical Engineers, Basic problems of prehension, movement and control of artificial limbs, Proceedings 1968–1969*, 1968;**183**(3J):54–59

Chapter 5
Hand assessment

5.1 Introduction

An engineer will design a new hand using a range of analytical and computer simulation methods. Components and sub-assemblies are constructed from the conceptual drawings and tested to see if they meet the required mechanical and electrical specifications. These tests vary in complexity. Mechanical testing can be achieved through cycling the component, e.g., counting the number of times a finger can be flexed and extended before it no longer functions. During these tests, weak components can be identified and replaced with better ones. Oscilloscopes and multimeters can measure and record electrical variables and parameters such as voltages, currents, resistances and inductances. Observing and analysing waveform data from a digital storage oscilloscope informs a designer of where component voltages, currents and power need adjustment or a major redesign is necessary. Once a design is deemed to be within the specifications, a hand needs to meet standards such as electromagnetic compatibility or EMC so that the electronic and electrical components do not radiate electromagnetic interference signals and also operate safely when there is some electromagnetic noise in the environment. But all of these physical testing and data analysis do not inform an engineer about the functionality of an artificial hand. Only by attaching it to a person and assessing its operation in practice can one hand be improved or be compared to another hand.

5.1.1 How can the function of a hand design be assessed?

An Oxford English Dictionary definition of 'function' is

> Activity; action in general, whether physical or mental. Of a person: Bearing, gestures.

Light proposed a general definition of functionality in the phrase 'suitability to task'. So what is required is a method that estimates the performance of a hand with respect to some physical action performed by a person. What is needed is a standardised, reliable and validated test (Table 5.1).

Table 5.1 Specification for a hand assessment

• Low cost	• Reliable (test–retest, inter-rater)
• Validated (criterion, content)	• Portable
• Time taken to carry out test less than half an hour	• Easy to manufacture
• Easy to use	• Minimise variability of physical components
• Applicable to a wide range of natural and artificial hands	• Standardised
• Self-administered	• Measurements are independent of the assessor

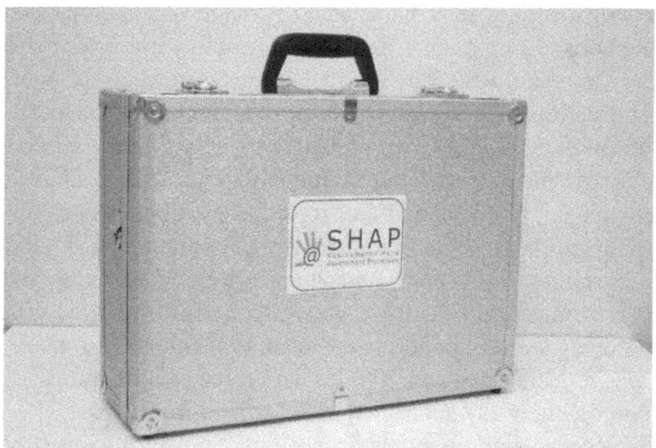

Figure 5.1 SHAP case

5.2 The Southampton Hand Assessment Procedure

The Southampton Hand Assessment Procedure (SHAP) consists of 12 abstract tests (6 lightweight and 6 heavyweight) and 14 activities of daily living (ADL) tests [1–3]. It is portable, and all the equipment fits neatly into a metal case (Figure 5.1). Figure 5.2 shows the abstract objects and Table 5.2 lists them. The objects are shown with the form board that has several functions. For the abstract test objects it is used to locate positions of the test objects on a flat surface (Figure 5.3). Figure 5.4 shows the ADL components and Table 5.3 lists them. The white side of the form board is shown in Figure 5.5, which is also used to locate components for some of the ADL tests. SHAP includes a timer so that the times recorded for each test are from tasks carried out by the person being assessed and do not include any reaction times or biases from the assessor. Also the procedure has been clinically validated. An overall score for the procedure is calculated from the times taken to carry out each of the 26 tests and is recorded out of 100. SHAP is used internationally to assess both natural and artificial hands [4–19].

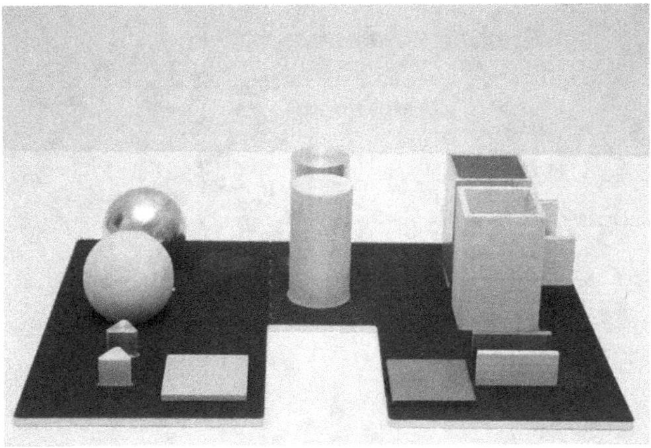

Figure 5.2 Abstract objects and the form board

Table 5.2 Abstract objects

		Light	Heavy
Tripod	Triangular prism	Balsa	Aluminium
Tip	Small thick plate	Balsa	Steel
Lateral	Square tube cup with side piece	Balsa	Aluminium
Power	Cylinder	Balsa	Aluminium
Spherical	Sphere	Balsa	Aluminium
Extension	Thick plate	Balsa	Steel

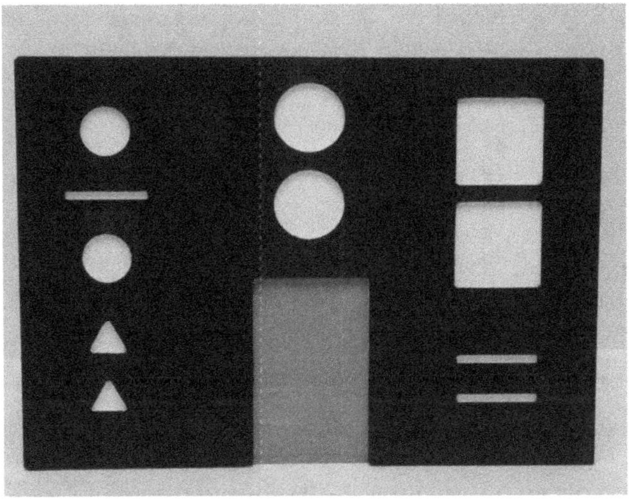

Figure 5.3 One side of the form board showing the locations of the abstract objects for each task

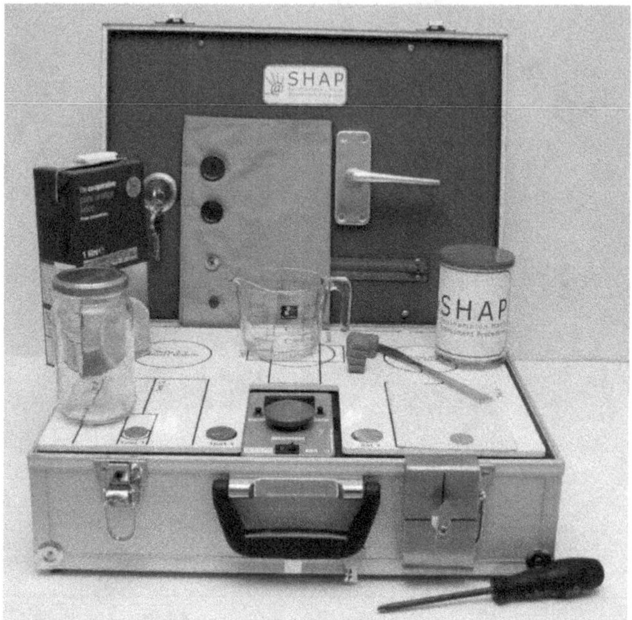

Figure 5.4 SHAP case opened showing the ADL components

Table 5.3 Activities of daily living

Number	Task	Classification of pattern
1	Pick up coins	Tip
2	Buttons	Tip and tripod
3	Food cutting	Tripod and power
4	Simulated page turning	Extension
5	Remove jar lid	Spherical
6	Pour water from jug	Lateral
7	Pour water from carton	Spherical
8	Move empty jar	Power
9	Move tray	Lateral and extension
10	Move full jar	Power
11	Rotate key 90 degrees	Tip and lateral
12	Open and close zip	Tip and lateral
13	Rotate door handle	Power
14	Rotate screw 90^0	Power

As an example of one of the tasks, Figures 5.6–5.11 shows a sequence of photographs for the assessment of the lightweight 'power' (cylinder) object.

5.2.1 Prehensile patterns

The postures of the hand are infinitely variable due to the high number of degrees of freedom in a natural hand anatomy. For SHAP, an economic number of classes

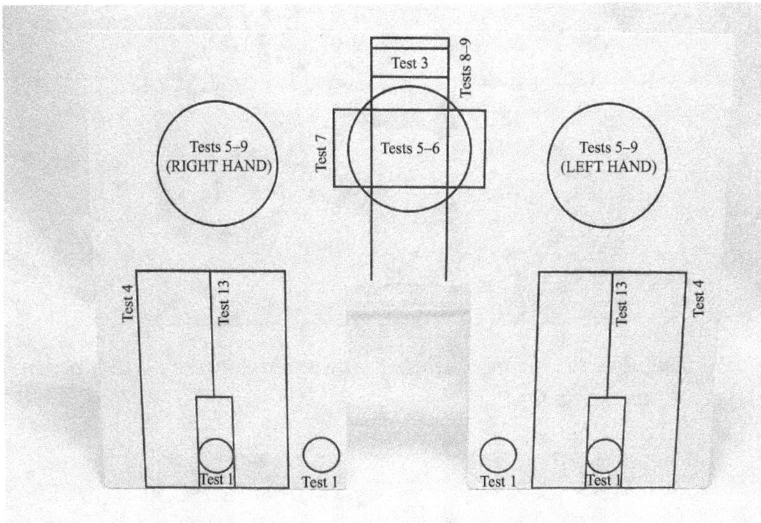

Figure 5.5 ADL side of the form board

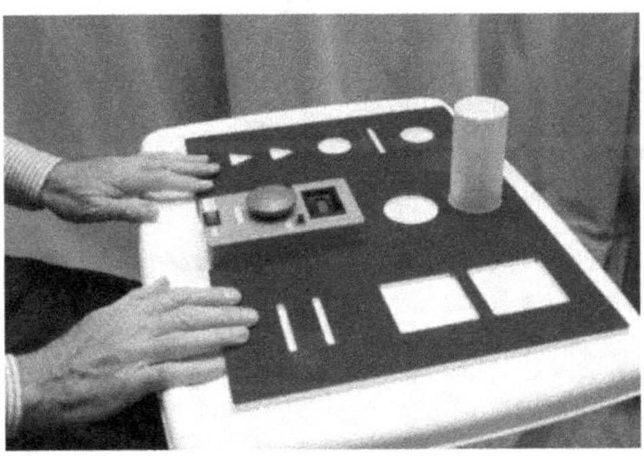

Figure 5.6 The person is seated at a table with their hands placed either side of the timer which is the grey box with the large central push button. The timer is set to zero

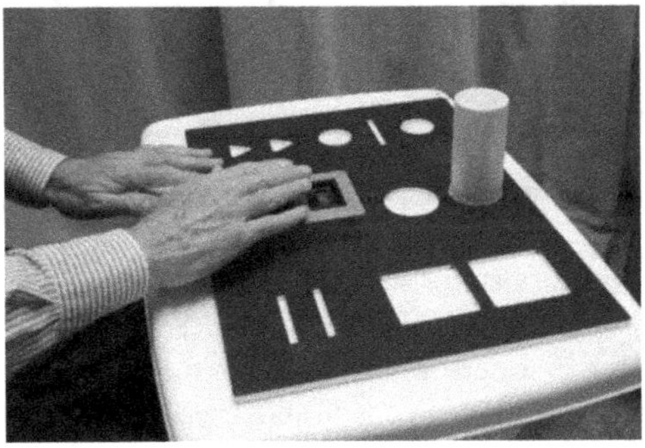

Figure 5.7 The timer is started by depressing the blue button

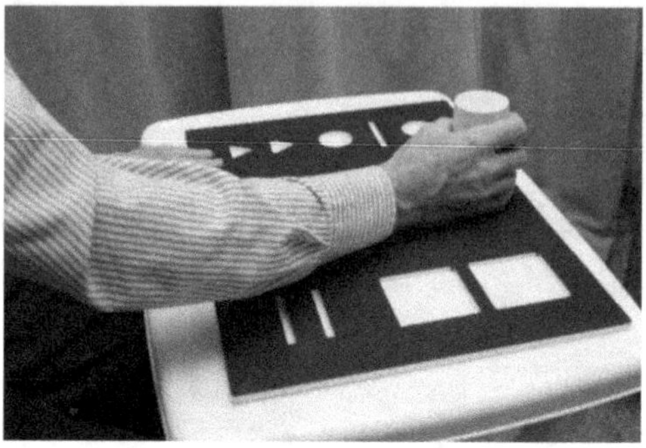

Figure 5.8 The object is gripped using a 'power' prehensile pattern at the back of the form board

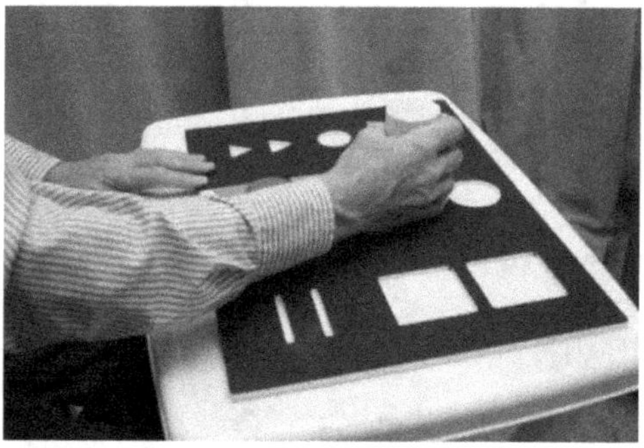

Figure 5.9 The 'power' object is moved to the second locating position on the form board

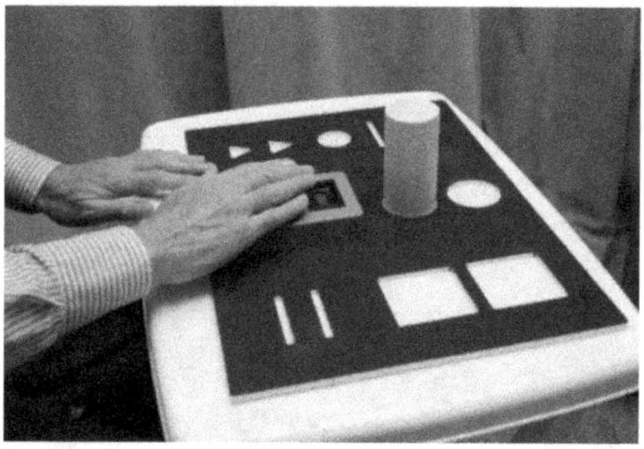

Figure 5.10 The timer is stopped

for classification of hand postures are six (Figure 5.12). The abstract objects are based on these six patterns (Table 5.4 and Figure 5.12). The light set are made of balsa wood, and therefore a person's hand forms the shape of the abstract posture and requires a light grip on an object (Table 5.4). The heavy set is made from metals, and therefore a firmer gasp is needed to move an object.

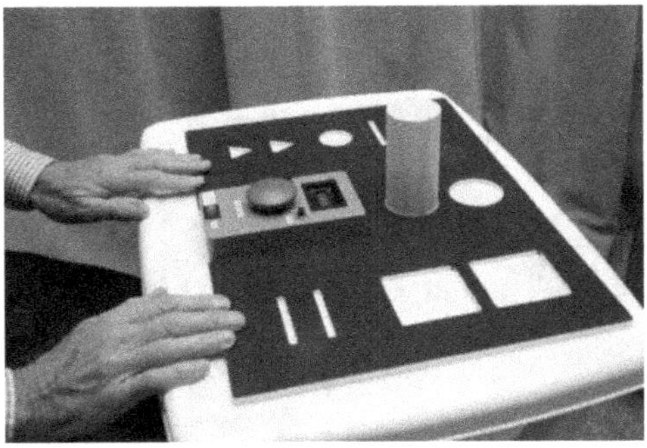

Figure 5.11 The hand is returned to the table

Table 5.4 Prehensile patterns

Tripod	Pulp of the index/middle fingers opposes that of the thumb
Tip	Tip of the thumb opposes that of one/two fingers
Lateral	Lateral side of the index finger opposes the pulp of the thumb
Power	All fingers are flexed into the palm
Spherical	Fingers and thumb are flexed and adducted. Thumb is rotated
Extension	Fingers and thumb are extended. Fingers are abducted in opposition to the thumb

5.3 Procedure

The person to be assessed is seated at a table with the task placed in front of them. The person starts the timer by depressing the large blue button on the grey timer box. The task is carried out and then the timer stopped, and the time taken to complete the task is recorded by the assessor. For the abstract test objects the form board is placed about 80 mm from the front of the table.

The white side of the form board is used for the ADL tests except for the last four tests where the components are located either at the back of the case (tests 11 key, 12 zip and 13 handle) or attached to the front of the case (test 14, rotate the screw by 90 degrees).

5.4 Calculations

One of the founding principles of SHAP was the ability to maintain consistent and transferrable outcome measures, which requires a standardised analysis of data. This principle has been achieved through one supplier of the kit, where a rigorous attention to the detail of manufacture for each part of the kit has been maintained as explained later. Then a normative set of scores was found by experimenting on people who were considered as representative of a prime set. This group of subjects were undergraduates with an age range of 18–25 years who did not have any physiological conditions of the upper limb. The set consists of times from 24 people.

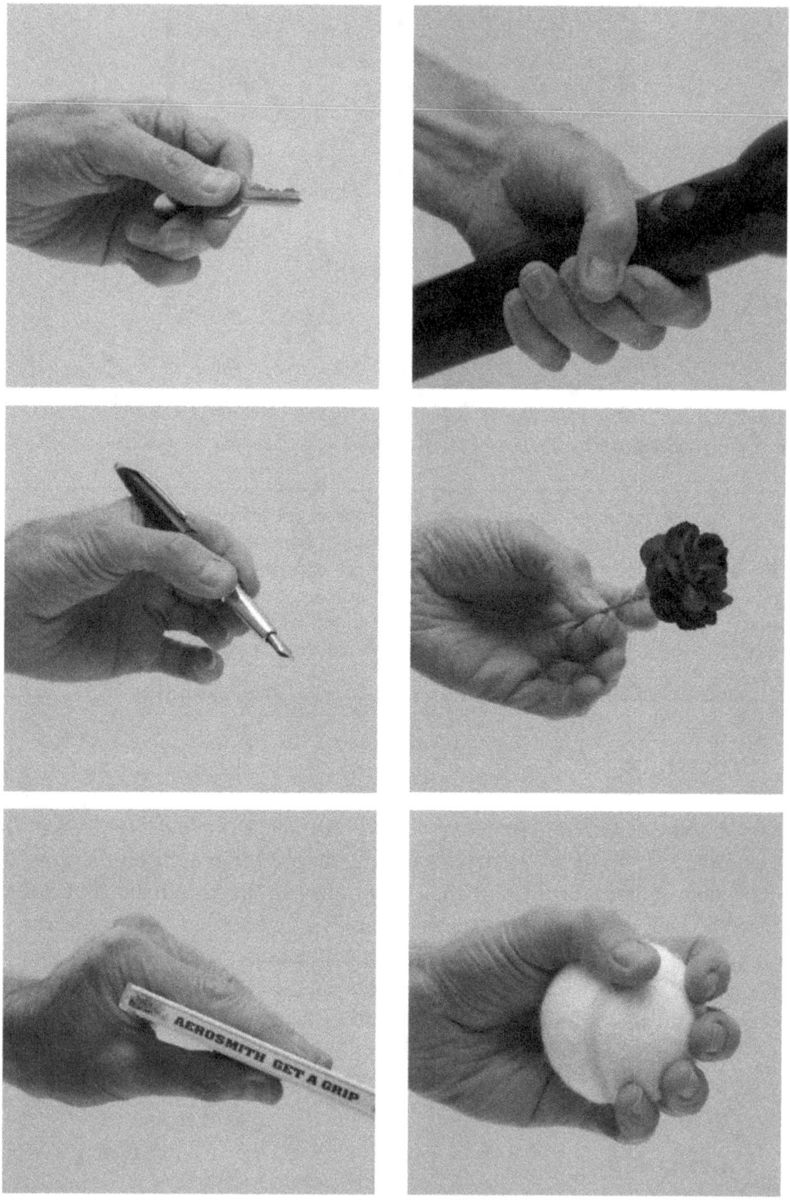

Figure 5.12 Prehensile patterns. From the left to right and top to bottom; lateral, power, tripod, tip, extension and spherical

For a pattern, j, the z score is calculated from the following equation.

$$z_j = \frac{t_j - \overline{t_{nj}}}{\sigma_{nj}} \tag{5.1}$$

where z_j is the score for prehensile pattern j, t_j is the person's time for pattern j, $\overline{t_{nj}}$ is the mean time in the normative group for pattern j and σ_{nj} is the standard deviation for the normative group.

The main SHAP score or index of functionality, IOF, is calculated from the Euclidean distance which is the squared distance in six dimensions representing the distance of all six prehensile patterns from the normative value.

$$d_e = \sqrt{\sum_{j=1}^{6} z_j^2} \tag{5.2}$$

where d_e is the Euclidean distance.

A person who achieves the same times as the mean of the normative group has a Euclidean distance of zero (5.1 and 5.2). This is set as a score of 100. People taking longer times than the normative group have positive Euclidean distances, and the IOF is rescaled down towards zero.

A person with an injury to their first finger may find that their time for the task with the tripod abstract object and other related ADL are lower than the normative times. Monitoring of any progress in their treatment can be achieved by recording the changes to both their IOF and a metric of their tripod IOF score. The tripod IOF is determined in a similar calculation to the overall IOF (5.1 and 5.2). Also IOF are calculated for the other five prehensile patterns.

5.5 Manufacture

The abstract objects are made from materials that are readily available. The lightweight ones are handcrafted into the various shapes from balsa wood sheets, planks, rods and blocks. A prism object is made from a square cross-sectioned rod of material using a dividing head, milling machine and lathe. The tip, lateral and extension are formed from thick sheets; the sides, walls, base and side handle of the lateral object are glued together. A power object is made from a square-sectioned length in a lathe. The most labour-intensive object to make is the sphere. These objects are carefully formed in a lathe from a block of wood with a square cross-section using emery papers in a range of different grades. The balsa wood for the lightweight objects in this application is durable provided that the wood is selected and bowed, soft and uneven-grained wood discarded.

The heavyweight objects are either handcrafted with standard workshop tools, a lathe or using a Computer Numerically Controlled (CNC) machine. An aluminium rod is shaped into a prism using a milling machine and lathe. Thick bars of steel and aluminium are manually formed into the tip and extension objects. An aluminium tube forms the main part of the lateral object; two screws are used to attach a handle to one of the side walls. The power object is manufactured from a round section of aluminium rod in a lathe. While the original spherical objects were made by hand from aluminium rod in a lathe, a more efficient method is to use a CNC machine.

All the abstract objects are made to exacting standards. The dimensions of each object are checked, so that their shape and mass are within tolerance.

The form board is made from a thick plastic cream sheet in a CNC machine and finished in blue baize on one side for placement of the abstract objects. It is covered on the other side with a stick-on transparent sheet to mark where some of the ADL parts are positioned. Four UK coins (2 p and 1 p) are used in the task of picking up and moving coins. A piece of folded cloth, backed by cardboard with four buttons is stitched together to make the button board. A rough cylinder of plasticine is cut with a table knife in the simulation of food cutting. Turning a page in a book is simulated by turning a rectangle of thin cardboard. A standard glass jar is used in the tasks of removing a jar lid, pouring water from a jug, pouring water from a carton, moving an empty jar and moving a full jar. The Pyrex jug has a unique shape with a handle shaped in a hook. A standard 1 L drinks carton is used in the task of pouring water into the jug. A spring and stop mechanism, attached to the back of a standard rim cylinder lock, is mounted on the red plastic back panel. This mechanism allows a key to be rotated clockwise through an angle of 90 degree against a small spring, simulating the resistance found when rotating an actual lock in a door. In the middle of the back panel is a zip mounted horizontally.

The resistance felt when rotating a door handle is simulated with a spring mechanism behind the back panel. The rotation of a screw by a screwdriver is simulated with an aluminium sheet bent in to a hook shape with a PTFE and aluminium insert. Some of the ADL parts are handmade from various materials but where a commercial component is used a careful choice has been made. Considering door handles, these are manufactured in a vast range and some are country specific. For example, North American handles tend to be round requiring a different grip pattern to that used in SHAP. The typed used in SHAP can be sourced in different styles; they can be left or right handed with the axis of rotation at the top, middle or bottom. Only one of these designs is specified for a SHAP kit.

Some ADL commercial parts are supplied in a standard form, e.g., rim cylinder locks, since they are designed to easily replace an existing lock in a door where the key needs to be changed. It is therefore possible to make a standard part for SHAP. However, some parts have more variability, e.g., the 1 L carton. On one occasion the red back panel was broken on its way through customs at an airport. Observations of the breakage indicated that the screwdriver had not been packed but been placed randomly in the case and then the lid forced to close the case. To overcome potential damage in future transits, a foam support is placed behind the whole panel to cushion any impact forces made by careless packing of the SHAP components and forcing the case closed.

5.6 Standardisation

The measurement of a physical quantity such as length (metre), mass (kilogram) or time (second) is encompassed in internationally agreed standards. Consider a simple example of the measurement of the diameter of the power heavyweight object.

A typical digital calliper will measure the diameter to a precision of 0.01 mm (0.0005″) and accuracy of ±0.02 mm (0.001″). This implies that the calliper has been calibrated against the standard metre. The definition of a metre has changed with the passing of time but it was defined in the ninth century as the distance between two lines of an alloy bar of platinum and iridium held in France at the melting point of ice.

What has all of these standards to do with SHAP? The unit of SHAP has been derived from a set of normative times from 24 people. These times represent an equivalent distance between two lines on the alloy bar kept in France. Any SHAP score from an assessed person using a SHAP kit is in effect being compared to this standard. To change the standard times or adjust the values in some arbitrary way is a bad idea as then a comparison of the SHAP score derived from the standard in one study cannot be compared to that obtained from a different study using a different standard. If the standard for the unit of measurement has been changed, then the procedure is not calibrated.

Through maintained tight control over the component manufacture, each kit has the same physical properties and adopting a standardised analysis of times to form SHAP scores then ensures a consistent and uniform procedure.

5.7 Reliability and validity

SHAP has been evaluated for giving consistent and reliable IOF scores by testing a control group of three people with three assessors. The test–retest and inter-rater reliability were at the 95% confidence level. The outcome measures were found to be reliable for a single assessor that is the test–retest evaluation and with multiple assessors that is the inter-rater reliability.

SHAP was assessed for validity by a panel of clinical professionals consisting of physiotherapists and occupational therapists. The panel gave feedback of the technique and recommendation of improvements implemented.

5.8 Physical process

In any assessment of upper limb functionality or any other investigation into the movement of the musculoskeletal system, fundamental classical physics as demonstrated by Sir Isaac Newton is applicable. Picking up an object and placing it somewhere else requires an input of energy from contracting muscles. An object held in a hand experiences a gravitational force, and some energy is dissipated in maintaining the object grip. The object may also be raised and will have potential energy in proportion to the height that it is raised. Some energy is recoverable since muscles have elasticity when they are stretched in a similar way as a spring can be used to store energy. Movement of the upper limb with the hand holding an object requires a complex and three-dimensional analysis of the kinetics and kinematics of the system.

To illustrate the interplay between energy, acceleration, velocity, distance and time, consider a simple analysis of rectilinear motion where an object is moved in a straight line and is not in a gravitational field. A constant acceleration is applied to a 500 g object (Figure 5.13) where the force is constant at 49.05 N. It is then decelerated with the same force. The velocity ramps up and then down (Figure 5.14). The corresponding distance moved is nonlinear (Figure 5.15) while the energy stored

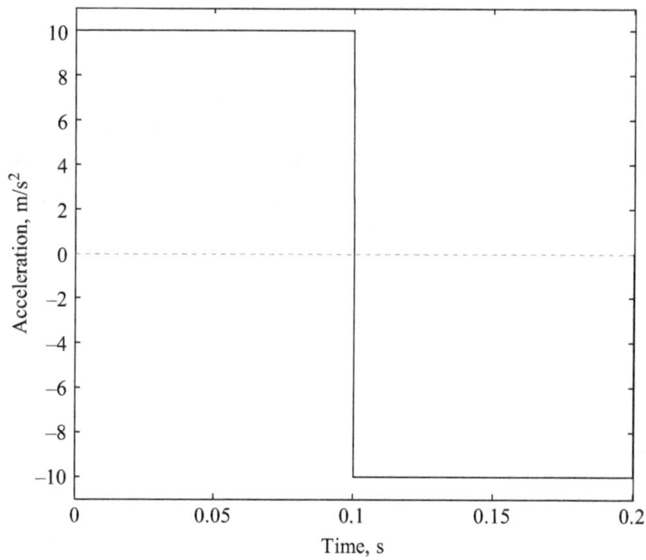

Figure 5.13 Acceleration

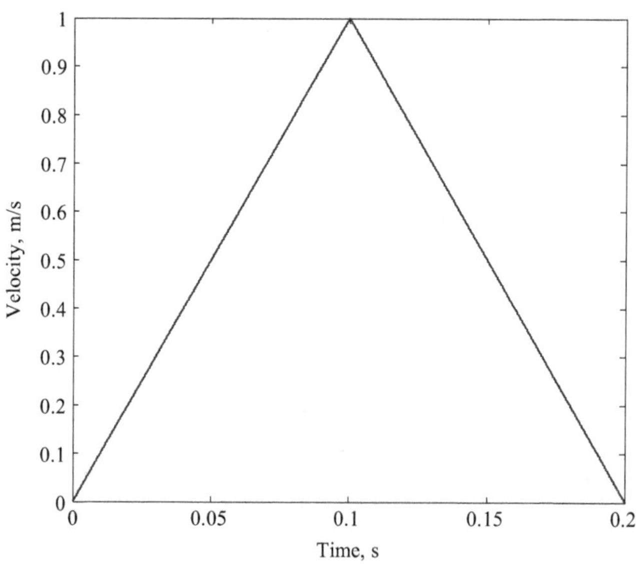

Figure 5.14 Velocity

and released from the object is also nonlinear (Figure 5.16). However the input of energy required is different (Figure 5.17). This analysis demonstrates the nonlinear nature of the energy from muscles in moving an object from one place to the next as would be found in any functional assessment.

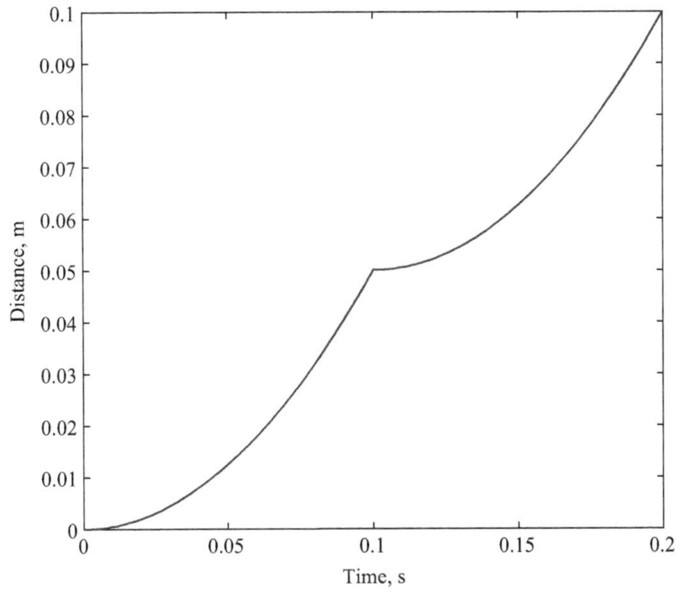

Figure 5.15 Distance

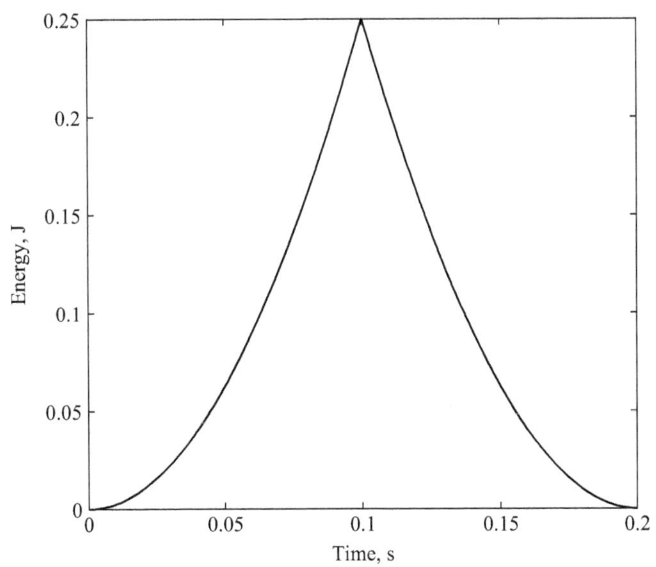

Figure 5.16 Energy stored in the object

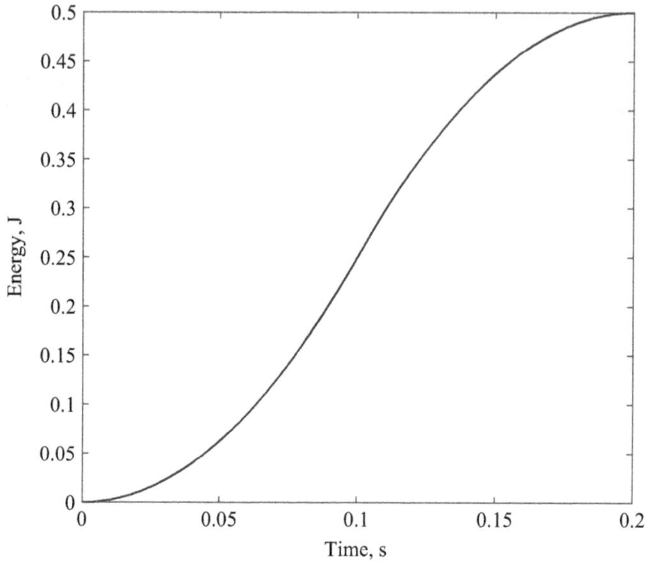

Figure 5.17 Energy needed to accelerate and decelerate the object, i.e., energy from the muscles

For a constant acceleration, A

$$\ddot{x} = A \tag{5.3}$$

The velocity is

$$\dot{x} = At \tag{5.4}$$

The distance travelled is

$$x = A\frac{t^2}{2} \tag{5.5}$$

And the energy, E, is

$$E = \frac{1}{2} m\dot{x}^2 \tag{5.6}$$

where the mass of the object is m.

Substituting the velocity equation into the energy equation

$$E = \frac{1}{2} mA^2t^2 \tag{5.7}$$

Under deceleration the force and acceleration are reversed, i.e., are negative. However, the equations have the same form as those for the acceleration as shown in the figures.

If the time taken to reach the peak velocity is T, then the peak energy stored in the object is

$$E = \frac{1}{2} m A^2 T^2 \tag{5.8}$$

But the same amount of energy is required to decelerate the object, so the input of energy from the muscles is

$$E = m A^2 T^2 \tag{5.9}$$

The distance at peak velocity, X, is

$$X = A \frac{T^2}{2} \tag{5.10}$$

or

$$A = X \frac{2}{T^2} \tag{5.11}$$

Substituting this equation into the energy equation and eliminating A,

$$E = \frac{4mX^2}{T^2} \tag{5.12}$$

Consider a pair of muscles accelerating a mass, held in a hand, and then decelerating it. The analysis shown above indicates that the energy put into the mass is inversely proportional to the square of the time taken (5.7). In a hand assessment, such as SHAP, the person being assessed is asked to move an object of mass, m, a fixed distance, X and the time is recorded, T. Plotting the variation of energy with time taken is shown in Figure 5.18. The analysis illustrates the non-linear nature of the motion of an object. In practice, a person moving an object, e.g., a heavy sphere, will use more than one muscle and more energy; the object will experience changes in potential energy as a result of being in the Earth's gravitational field; there will be rotation of the object and the motion will occur in three dimensions. Hence, the time taken is dependent on many factors. Also there will be the neurological delays in transmitting information around the person's body from sensors along neural pathways and to muscles to maintain grip forces or adjust the posture of the upper limb. There is experimental evidence that the wrist is rotated at constant velocity during movement of a sphere in one of the SHAP abstract object tasks. This result suggests that rather than the object being accelerated and decelerated as in Figure 5.13, there is a period in between acceleration and deceleration where there is no acceleration.

The parameters in the figures are typical for a person moving a heavy sphere in the SHAP task. In Figure 5.18 the energy required to move an object a set distance

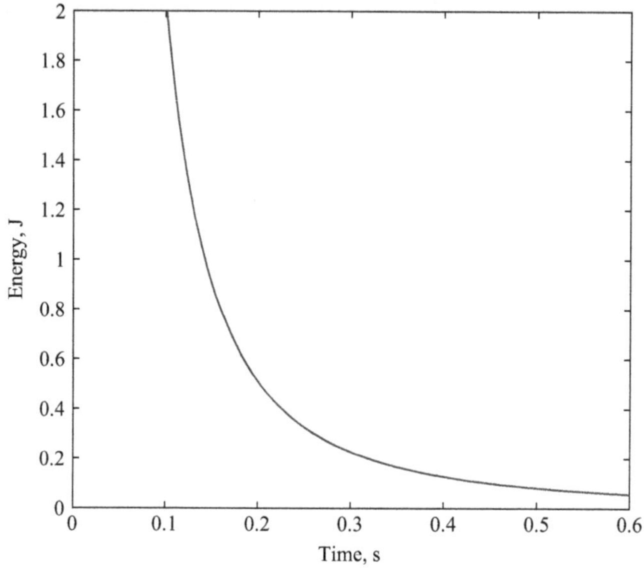

Figure 5.18 Energy input for moving an object (mass of 0.5 kg) a distance of 0.2 m

increases rapidly as the time taken to carry out the task shortens. This is shown by the sensitivity as the change in energy with time as

$$\frac{dE}{dT} = -\frac{4mX^2}{3T^3} \tag{5.13}$$

The time taken in any assessment for a person who can impart a large force on an object will not decrease very much if they reduce the force by 10% (towards the left side of Figure 5.18). Whereas a person whose time is slower than normal will show a larger increase in the time taken, if they reduce their effort by 10% (towards the right side of Figure 5.18).

5.9 Small SHAP

Relative to the effort put into the design and manufacture of adult hands, there has been little research and development of smaller hands for adults and in particular for children [20]. Some companies have reduced the size of their adult hand to accommodate the smaller person particularly for the female population. These hands fall into the category of hands for teenagers. The choice of a hand for a child is limited. As well as a need to evaluate current designs for children, a small SHAP kit is needed to evaluate future designs as well as being useful for testing the functionality of the diseased or injured hand.

With this in mind some progress has been made to meet this need. Starting with the abstract test objects, these can be scaled down but the question that needs

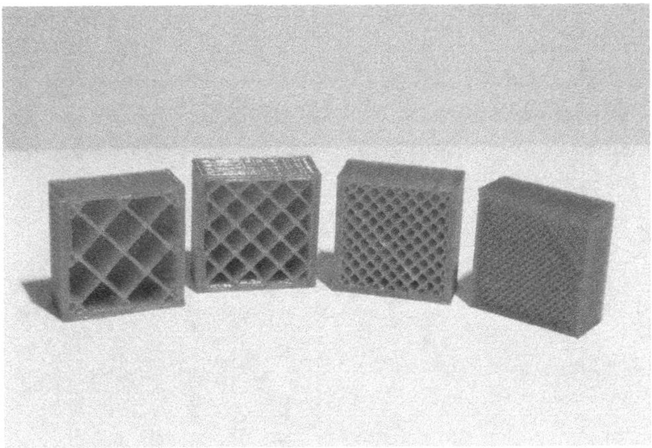

Figure 5.19 Cuboid objects with different internal structures made using 3D printing from PLA. Their dimensions are 2.52 × 2.48 × 1.11 cm with a volume of 6.92 cm^{-3}. The outer and inner walls have a mean thickness of 1.6 and 0.49 mm, respectively (ranges 1.26–1.83 mm and 0.45–0.53 mm). Sample 1 is at the left hand side and sample 4 at the right hand side

to be answered is by how much? At the smallest end of the spectrum is the 5-year old that may be sufficiently attentive to carry out a SHAP test, while at the other end is the 10-year old whose hand parameters such as finger length are sufficiently near to that of an adult that the present SHAP can be used.

An analysis of normal hand measurements for children from 4 to 7 years old has shown that there is a linear relationship between hand length, middle finger length, palm length and palm width with age. The average of these parameters with age ranges from 63% at 4 years to 73% at 7 years compared to that of an average adult hand (where 100% is the parameter value for an adult hand) [20]. At the smallest size, reducing the abstract test objects by two thirds, would seem an appropriate amount.

Consider the lightweight abstract test objects. The full-sized versions are made from balsa wood that has an average density of 0.15 g·cm^{-3} (range 0.1–0.2 g·cm^{-3}). The test objects with a reduction in dimensions could also be manufactured from balsa wood, but there are other materials that could be used, particularly polymers. The improvements made in 3D printing should lead to quicker manufacturing times and at a lower cost. ABS (Polyacrylonitrile–butadiene–styrene) has a density of 1.05 g·cm^{-3} that is denser by a factor of seven compared to balsa wood. Similarly PLA (polylactic acid–bipolymer) has a slightly higher density of 1.24 g·cm^{-3}; it is denser by a ratio of 8.3:1 compared to balsa wood. In order to lower the mass of an object to that of one made from balsa wood requires making hollow structures if plastic materials are used. Figure 5.19 shows four cuboids with the same dimensions where internally there are supporting walls. By reducing the rigidity of the object, a saving in mass of more than 50% can be made. However, the orientation of a

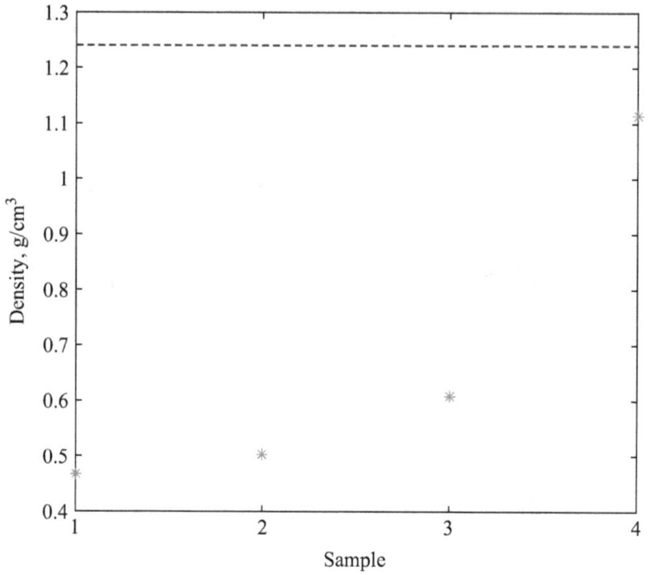

Figure 5.20 Density of PLA sample cuboids with a dotted horizontal line for the solid density of 1.24 g·cm^{-3}. These data are from the samples shown in Figure 5.19, sample 1 is at the left hand side and sample 4 at the right hand side

supporting internal structure results in an object that does not have isomorphic properties, and it will have a higher tensile strength in one direction. Also as the object is made from layers of material, the physical properties in the plane (x, y directions) of the layers are different when compared to those at right angles to the plane (vertical z direction). For some 3D printed objects, the tensile strength is higher at right angles to the plane of the layers.

The density of the four cuboid samples are shown in Figure 5.20 and the relative densities compared to solid PLA are shown in Figure 5.21. For the particular software controlling the 3D printer, the maximum density setting is for sample 4 which is 90% of the solid material.

As an example, consider the lightweight sphere that is to be reduced in diameter. The volume is

$$\text{volume} = \frac{4}{3}\pi\left(\frac{d}{2}\right)^3 \tag{5.14}$$

So the mass will also vary as the cube of the diameter. The masses as a function of the diameter, for the four samples, are shown in Figure 5.22. A sphere made from the lowest density sample is more than 50% heavier than that made from balsa wood.

Parts of an artificial hand could also be made using internal structures to reduce the mass, but some materials are not suitable, e.g., PLA is biodegradable.

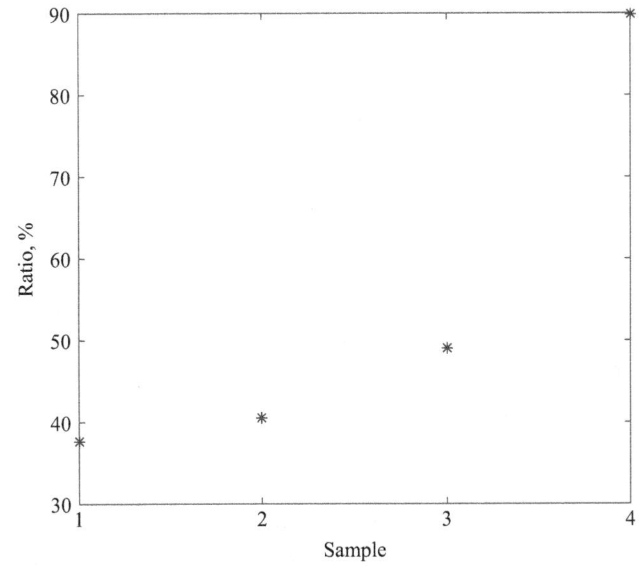

Figure 5.21 Density of the cuboid samples relative to the PLA solid density of 1.24 g·cm^{-3}. These data are from the samples shown in Figure 5.19, sample 1 is at the left hand side and sample 4 at the right hand side

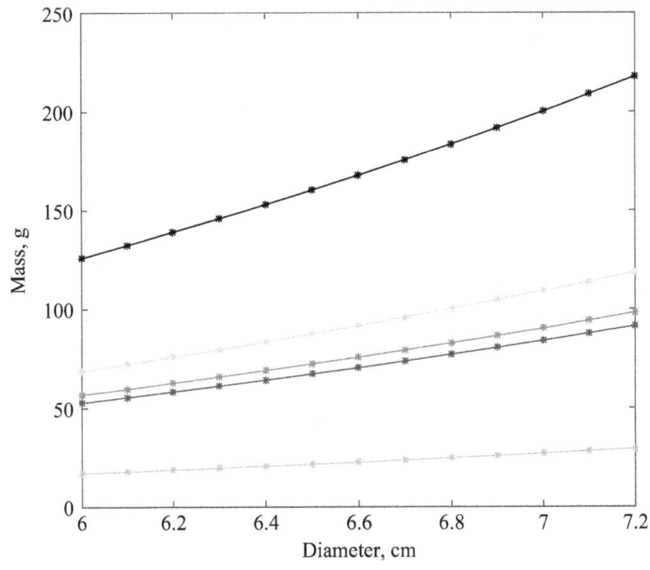

Figure 5.22 Comparing the mass of a lightweight sphere for four densities with different internal structures based on the samples of PLA shown in Figure 5.19. From top to bottom, the curves are for samples 4, 3, 2 and 1, respectively. For comparison, the lower curve shows the mass for a balsa sphere with a density of 0.15 g·cm^{-3}

5.10 Summary

The assessment of natural or artificial hand function is wide reaching. Any procedure should satisfy a set of main criteria; reliability (inter-rater), standardised equipment, validated, portable and standardised metrics. All of these criteria are encompassed in the SHAP. The movement of an abstract test object or the manipulation of an everyday object used in ADL requires coordination of the neuromuscular system and can be related back to the time taken to carry out the task. The underlying physics and control of a moving object can provide evidence and give clues as to the way that the assessment is performed by a person. Making a smaller version of SHAP for the assessment of children requires careful consideration of materials especially for the design of the lightweight abstract test objects.

References

1 Light C. M. *An Intelligent Hand Prosthesis and Evaluation of Pathological and Prosthetic Hand Function*, PhD thesis, University of Southampton, 2000

2 Light C. M., Chappell P. H., and Kyberd P. J. 'Establishing a standardized clinical assessment tool of pathologic and prosthetic hand function: normative data, reliability, and validity', *Archives of Physical Medicine and Rehabilitation*, 2002;**83**:776–783

3 Light C. M., Chappell P. H., Kyberd P. J., and Ellis B. S. 'A critical review of functionality assessment in natural and prosthetic hands', *British Journal of Occupational Therapy*, 1999;**62**:7–12

4 Aszmann O. C., Roche A. D., Salminger S., *et al.* 'Bionic reconstruction to restore hand function after brachial plexus injury: a case series of three patients', *The Lancet*, 2015;**385**(9983):2183–2189

5 Dalley S. A., Bennett D. A., and Goldfarb M. 'Functional assessment of the vanderbilt multigrasp myoelectric hand: a continuing case study', *Engineering in Medicine and Biology Society (EMBC), 2014 36th Annual International Conference of the IEEE*, 2014:6195–6198

6 Hermannsson L. M. N., Andrén M., and Johansson D. 'Swedish normative data for the Southampton Hand Assessment Procedure – SHAP', *Myoelectric Controls Conference MEC '14 – Redefining the Norm*, University of New Brunswick, Fredericton, Canada, August 19–22, 2014, 86

7 Fougner A. L., Stavdahl Ø., and Kyberd P. J. 'System training and assessment in simultaneous proportional myoelectric prosthesis control', *Journal of NeuroEngineering and Rehabilitation*, 2014;**11**:75

8 Vasluian E., Bongers R. M., Reinders-Messelink H. A., Dijkstra P. U., and van der Sluis C. K. 'Preliminary study of the Southampton Hand Assessment Procedure for children and its reliability', *BMC Musculoskeletal Disorders*, 2014;**15**:199

9 van der Niet O., Bongers R. M., and van der Sluis C. K. 'Functionality of i-LIMB and i-LIMB pulse hands: case report', *Journal of Rehabilitation Research & Development*, 2013;**50**(8):1123–1128

10 Kyberd P. J. 'The influence of control format and hand design in single axis myoelectric hands: assessment of functionality of prosthetic hands using the Southampton Hand Assessment Procedure', *Prosthetics and Orthotics International*, 2011;**35**(3):285–293

11 Van der Niet Otr O., Reinders-Messelink H. A., Bongers R. M., Bousema H., and van der Sluis C. 'The i-LIMB hand and the DMC plus hand compared: a case report', *Prosthetics and Orthotics International*, 2011;**34**(2):216–220

12 Issa A. R., Lusk C. P., Dubey R., Highsmith M. J., and Maitland M. E. 'Crossed four-bar mechanism for improved prosthetic grasp', *Journal of Rehabilitation Research and Development*, 2009;**46**(8):1011–1020

13 Kyberd P. J., Murgia A., Gasson M., *et al.* 'Case studies to demonstrate the range of applications of the Southampton Hand Assessment Procedure' *British Journal of Occupational Therapy*, 2009;**72**(5):212–218

14 Metcalf C. D., Woodward H., Wright V., Chappell P. H., Burridge J. H., and Yule V. T. 'Changes in hand function with age and normative unimpaired scores when measured with the Southampton Hand Assessment Procedure', *British Journal of Hand Therapy*, 2008;**13**(3):79–83

15 Metcalf C. D. *The Relationship Between Movement and Function of the Wrist and Hand: A Clinically Focused Kinematic Study*, PhD thesis, University of Southampton, 2008

16 Adams J., Metcalf C. D., Macleod C., *et al.* 'Three dimensional functional motion analysis of silver ring splints in rheumatoid arthritis', *Rheumatology: British Society of Rheumatology Annual Meeting*, 2008;**47**(Suppl 2):ii154–ii155

17 Metcalf C. D., Adams J. A., Burridge J. H., Yule V. T., and Chappell P. H. 'A review of clinical upper limb assessments within the framework of the WHO ICF', *Musculoskeletal Care*, 2007;**5**(3):160–173

18 Murgia A. *A Gait Analysis Approach to the Study of Upper Limb Kinematics Using Activities of Daily Living*, PhD thesis, University of Reading, 2005

19 Cary I. and Adams J. 'A comparison of dominant and non-dominant hand function in both right and left handed individuals using the Southampton Hand Assessment Procedure (SHAP)', *British Journal of Hand Therapy*, 2003;**8**(1):4–10

20 Redman T. R. *The Design of a Myoelectrically Controlled Hand with Multiple Actuators for Children*, PhD thesis, University of Southampton, 2016

Chapter 6
Future directions

An outline of the engineering requirements for a prosthetic hand has been described in this book where the techniques and ideas presented are also applicable to robotic hands. Of all the components that form the system of an artificial hand, it is perhaps the algorithms, sensors and the processing of signals that will play an increasing role to improve the functionality of advanced hand designs [1–10].

The new developments in 3-D printing (additive manufacturing) allow for custom-made designs, modular components and low cost in the development of designs. However, the polymer-based materials have non-isometric properties and can be relatively weak compared to blocks of materials that are machined into the desired shape. Also if a high tolerance is required, then a 3-D printed component may lack the precision required. This technology has seen considerable development in the recent years and opens up the possibility of low cost and modular component design. Further developments, especially using low-density metals, will greatly enhance the durability of future prosthetics.

The cognitive burden placed on the wearer of an artificial upper limb will make it unusable, unless some simple control scheme is adopted to overcome this limitation. Information and signals from better sensors will drive the controller into making precise and automatic movements. More sophisticated mechanisms that seek to enhance the life-like appearance and function of a hand add unwanted mass and complexity. Future designs will need to address these problems, and it may be that a simple but novel idea will be seen as much more useful in everyday activities.

Materials science is a driving influence in prosthetic design. The density of an aluminium alloy, such as 6061 used in aircraft structures, is about 2.7 $g{\cdot}cm^{-1}$ and represents the upper bound for useful materials to be used in prosthetics. Materials that use polymers have about half the density of metal alloys but need to be mechanically robust with good tensile strength and resistance to abrasion. Also they need to be resistant to humid environments as plastics can change dimensions by as much as 10% when they absorb or release water vapour. Recent research into the addition of fillers in plastic materials may enhance the existing mechanical and electrical properties for prosthetic applications. Adding small amounts of nano-particles, such as carbon nanotubes and graphene, turn an insulating polymer into a conductor that can be used as a resistance strain gauge. Adding silica (silicon dioxide) particles to silicone can increase the tensile strength of a glove while retaining its elastic properties. It is necessary to observe safety handling procedures when adding nanoparticles to a polymer, as the particles may damage the respiratory system if inhaled and the longer term effects are not be known. Furthermore, the materials should conform to the appropriate mandatory regulation for medical devices as some of the components may be in contact with a skin surface.

An artificial sense of touch requires suitable sensors on the hand but also some method of processing the information and coding it into the natural sensory system. This connection may take the form of electrically stimulating the afferent sensory nerves requiring an invasive procedure. Alternatively the skin surface can be mechanically vibrated. This method is not new but recently there has been renewed interest in developing this technique, making use of scientific and technical developments. One method uses a small DC motor with an eccentric mass and can be used to create vibrations at about 250 Hz that are at the peak response of natural sensors below the surface of the skin [6, 7, 10, 11].

To increase functionality requires the addition of more actuators. Present designs are restricted by their high mass relative to the mass limit of the whole hand as explained in an earlier chapter. Increased power and torque of an electromechanical device with reduced size and mass from new technology, be it some novel technique or simply improvements to motor design, will greatly enhance any new artificial hand.

Sensors that meet the demanding mechanical and electrical specifications required for an artificial hand will continue to be developed. As well as being able to function with existing alloy materials, there will be a demand to work with lightweight materials such as polymers. The latter is potentially more difficult if integration of sensors into the structure of a hand is required since the processing of polymer sensors occurs at lower temperatures. Stainless steel can withstand temperature of 800°C whereas polymers are polymerised at much lower temperatures up to 300°C. New techniques, using different combinations of fillers in plastic materials to design new force slip and texture sensors will be under development. Information from these sensors could be sent wirelessly to the clinic and industry to monitor and record usage and faults (The Internet of Things).

References

1 Ahmad S. A. and Chappell P. H. 'Artificial prehension and the detection of object slip', *11th World Congress on Medical Physics & BioMedical Engineering*, Munich, Germany, 2009

2 Ahmad S. A. and Chappell P. H. 'Development of electromyographic control system based on pattern recognition for prosthetic hand application', *International Conference on Signal Processing and Pattern Recognition and Applications*, Innsbruck, Austria, 17–19 February, 2009, 120–125

3 Ahmad S. A. and Chappell P. H. 'Surface EMG classification using moving approximate entropy and fuzzy logic for prosthesis control', *Myoelectric Controls Conference MEC '08*, University of New Brunswick, Fredericton, Canada, 13–15 August, 2008, 136–139

4 Ahmad S. A. and Chappell P. H. 'Surface EMG classification using moving approximate entropy', *IEEE IET UTP International Conference on Intelligent and Advanced Systems*, Kuala Lumpur, Malaysia, November 2007, 1163–1167
5 Redman T., Sims T., Chappell P., *et al.* 'The design of a myoelectrically controlled hand with multiple actuators for five-year old children', *Myoelectric Controls Conference MEC '11 Raising the standard*, University of New Brunswick, Fredericton, Canada, 14–19 August, 2011, 83–86
6 Mohamad Hanif, Noor H. H., Chappell P. H., Cranny A., and White N. M. 'Surface texture detection with artificial fingers', *37th Annual International Conference of the IEEE Engineering in Medicine and Biology Society*, MiCo, Milano Conference Centre, Milano, Italy, 25–29 August, 2015, 4
7 Mohamad Hanif, Noor H. H., Chappell P. H., White N. M., and Cranny A. 'Development of vibrotactile sensory feedback for prosthetic hand users', *IASTED International Conference Biomedical Engineering (BioMed 2014),* Zurich, Switzerland, 23–25 June, 2014, 294–301
8 Muridan N., Chappell P. H., Cranny A., and White N. M. 'Texture sensor for a prosthetic hand', *Eurosensors XXIV*, Linz, Austria, 6–8 September, 2010, B3L-D, 1–4
9 Muridan N. and Chappell P. H. 'Detection of slip from multiple sites in an artificial finger', *Sensors and Their Applications XV*, Heriot-Watt University, Edinburgh, 5–7 October, 2009, 5–7
10 Chappell P. H., Muridan N., Mohamad Hanif, Noor H. H., Cranny A., and White N. M. 'Sensing texture using an artificial finger and a data analysis based on the standard deviation', *IET Science Measurement and Technology*, ISSN 1751-882, 2015, 1–9
11 Mohamad Hanif, Noor H. H., *Sensory feedback for artificial hands*, PhD thesis, University of Southampton, Southampton, UK, 2016

Index

www.ingramcontent.com/pod-product-compliance
Lightning Source LLC
LaVergne TN
LVHW011804200926
848484LV00003B/777

* 9 7 8 1 7 8 5 6 1 1 5 4 4 *